LOSING

WEIGHT

WITHOUT

LOSING YOUR

MIND

TABLE OF CONTENTS

To begin, I wish to express sincere appreciation to my students and clients who have allowed me to work with them to help become healthier. Thank you all for sharing your stories, your history, your sweat, your tears, and your joy, and for allowing me to be a part of it all. You are the reason I can write this all down. Thank you for the gift of your time, your honesty, and willingness to embark on a journey with me.

I have spent decades working in the health field, specifically with people wanting to change their outcome by changing their bodies. Over 3 decades, I have earned two doctorate degrees, I've taught anatomy, kinesiology, physiology, and exercise science at University, and I've owned two successful health centers. I am a health educator, medically based clinical hypnotherapist and psychotherapist, fitness professional, nutrition coach, weight loss specialist, and natural health practitioner. All of that to say that it was never really about a title I held, but it was more about whether I could actually help another human being find peace and appreciation with their bodies, which leads to better health. For me, that was the real reward.

In regards to weight loss, I have personally worked with thousands of people at this point, and it has helped me to form the distinct opinion that while there are plenty of ways to lose weight, the only way to truly *resolve* the issue is to look at the *whole* picture…the *whole* person, then approach the process with complete and utter honesty.

The human body has everything it needs to function well, to lose weight and maintain a healthy weight without pills, surgeries, or gimmicks. Typical weight loss "diets" are based upon deprivation, which can be a miserable experience with an extraordinarily high failure rate. Why do that to yourself? Why do that when there's a better, healthier, and more natural way? Isn't it time we learn to love, appreciate, and work with our bodies in a way that empowers our bodies and our minds to change in a positive and lasting way? It's time to stop the excuses, the crazy diets, the unnecessary medical interventions, and all of the other modes of nonsense that plagues the weight

1

loss industry and robs people of their time, their money, and even their hopes. It's time to tune into your *self*…your whole self. It's time to get in touch with your body and your mind in a way that is harmonious and beautifully honest. This process is about understanding and action. This is about breaking the weight loss struggle cycle and working with your body from a new perspective. It's about learning about *you* and what *your* particular body needs. We are all different. Your key to weight loss is specific to you.

This book is intended to take the reader to the very core of the issue and investigate what it *really* takes to achieve a healthy, leaner body for a lifetime. This isn't about a diet or a temporary fix. It's about creating greater awareness and learning how to work with your body and your mind in such a way that the body transforms itself into its healthiest version. It's important to learn how to understand *your* body's specific needs. You are in individual, and your needs are highly specific to you!

This journey is about working with your body at a deep and honest level, while finding balance in that very real world that you live in. It's about real people, with real bodies. It is a natural, logical, sensible, long-term lifestyle approach to overall health and well-being, which includes a healthy body weight. We don't need to try to trick or manipulate our bodies to lose weight. We just need to understand how our bodies work…honestly, without any manipulation of scientific data to try to convince you to buy into some false diet plan.

This is about using all parts of your mind to help your body. You are an intelligent being living in a brilliantly complex body that is constantly changing. Your mind and your thoughts are a part of the process! Steer your direction! Create your new self! You are more powerful than perhaps you were aware of. It's time to be fully aware. You have the power to create the healthiest version of you possible.

This is about love. It's about being willing to love yourself enough to make changes. It's about recognizing that taking the time to take care of yourself isn't selfish, it's generous.

The body is a wonderfully complex machine that's operating on some reasonably simple guidelines. It WANTS to be healthy. All it needs is what it needs. So, what does it need? Let's begin this journey and find out.

READ THIS AGAIN

It's time to tune into your SELF.

You are more powerful than perhaps you were aware of.

You have the power to create the healthiest you.

This is about love.

CALORIES IN, CALORIES OUT. RIGHT?

Just Do the Math

There are 3500 calories in a pound. So in theory, if you eat 3500 less calories than normal and keep everything else the same for a week, then by the end of the week you should lose one pound. Alternatively, you could also choose to eat the same as always, but burn an extra 3500 calories in activity and you would also lose a pound. Sounds pretty straight forward and simple, doesn't it? Then why does losing weight seem so hard? Perhaps it's because that while the math may be right, people aren't nearly as predictable as a math problem. This is why theories and text-book answers are only partially right, and also explains why people get so frustrated when they try to lose weight based on a generic formula. You are unique, and your body will respond in its own unique way.

The Math Works but the Textbook is Wrong

Is _your_ body a perfect specimen of a textbook human body? No flaws? No medications? No disease? No trauma? No issues? No imperfect DNA? No metabolic issues as a result from previous dieting? Are you also at your physical prime from a physiological perspective, around the age of 25? If you answered YES to these questions, then you just _might_ be an example of "text-book" potential. Congratulations! If however you answered NO to one or more of those questions (like most of us), you might find that little 3500 calorie trick to be a bit more elusive.

But wait, there is still more to it. We also need to find out if you have a perfect life to go with it. No stress? No worries? No time restraints? No emotional, financial, work or relationship issues? If you pass these questions off, then again, that 3500 calorie drop will fix things right up and you will lose that pound! Oh, but you need to be rather predictable too. You basically need to have the same caloric expenditure and input day after day so that

3500 calorie deficit will equal a whole, entire pound. So now what do you think? Do you have a perfect body, with a perfect and almost robotically routine life? If so, then the theory works and you probably don't actually need to read this book.

If however, this is not the case and you are like most of us who inhabit a body with some less-than-so-called "perfect" textbook qualities and/or you also live a life with ups, downs, and challenges because you are a *real* human being… then you are going to find that "calories in, calories out" theory to be a bit more complex. Soon it all starts to feel as though that "lose 3500 calories to lose a pound" thing is really the brain child of some evil mathematician-nutritionist type who was good at formulas but not so good at the practical application of such things.

The math formula has been tested using crazy foods to achieve/prove "results". Mark Haub, a Kansas State University professor ate Twinkies, chips, sugary cereals, and cookies every three hours, instead of meals. He continued to exercise and used a reduce calorie formula to lose weight and he lost weight. This same theory has been used with a variety of fast food restaurants by others and it's been the focus of a few documentaries. So does this mean that a person can eat garbage and lose weight? Sure. Does this mean that a person can eat junk and feel good and be healthy? Not really. We are talking about different things here.

Most diets, even crazy ones, will "work" but they don't actually *work*. They don't actually create a healthier person, with a healthier relationship with food and their body. But there's something to be said about the junk food diet experiments. It does make a point that perhaps we don't have to be "perfect" in order to be successful. In fact, maybe the pursuit of perfection is what got us into this head game.

So is the formula right? In theory…yes. In practice…not so much. In fact, sometimes calorie reduction totally backfires and cause weight gain! There are so many factors that need to be accounted for, particularly if you want long- term results.

What really works? It's not a formula or a number. It's about understanding *your* body's specific needs and responding to them. This is *personal*.

READ THIS AGAIN

You are unique, and your body will respond in its own unique way.

THE TRUTH

What's The Trick?

There's no trick really. There are however some basic realities that need to be considered if weight loss is a goal. Here are a few thoughts to get you started:

1. Your body is not a textbook example.

2. Your body is unique and you must tune into your unique self.

3. Stop blaming your body. You are not the victim of your biology. Everyone *can* lose weight but not everyone does. Those that don't lose weight *don't* actually take the right steps. Sometimes, those that do lose weight, *do or do not* take the right steps. Those that lose weight and keep it off, *do* take the right steps.

4. Some weight loss is real. Some weight loss is false or just temporary. You get to decide which weight loss you want. Although in my opinion, temporary action doesn't make much sense. But you get to decide what you are ready for.

5. There is no easy "magic" trick to losing weight. It takes change, determination, knowledge, consistency, and effort.

6. If you lose weight fast, that's actually a problem, not a goal.

7. *You* are responsible for your weight; not your personal trainer, not your nutritionist, not your hypnotist, not your doctor, not your spouse, not your parents, not your family, not your friends. *(An exception to this is if you are a child who is subject to living in a household that does not support good health, in which case it's the adult's responsibility.)*

8 Genetics are *not* a reason or an excuse to be fat. You may come from a family who is shaped like a pear (or an apple, or whatever shape your family tends to be), but you can still be a healthy pear shape (or a healthy apple shape, or whatever shape your family tends to be). Genetics only partially determine where your body likes to *store fat*, not whether or not you actually have excess fat to store. That is your choice. (Read point #7 again).

9. It's a simple path, not an easy one.

10. Your body is *YOURS*. Own it.

There are many truths and realities that come up as we move through this process, and together we will work through them one by one.

The weight loss industry is a multi-billion dollar business for a reason. Sadly, most of it is based off misleading consumers in order to make a profit. Consumers are bombarded with information about the latest diets, exercises, gimmicks, videos, pills, shakes, pre-packaged foods, protein bars, patches, surgeries, and so on, often with a shred of truth attached to make it all seem valid when in reality, it's probably not, at least not for long-term solutions. What the weight loss industry is lacking in is *the truth*…the *whole truth*. The truth is that you already have the tools you need to be successful! The problem is that most people don't know how to use those tools, don't want to put forth the effort, or have been so misled that they aren't sure what is right or wrong anymore.

As we move though this journey, we will be looking at things from a biological, physiological, psychological, and scientific perspective, rather than a "diet" perspective. This will allow you to filter out the nonsense and can help you to work with your body on a whole new level, as well as determine what your specific needs are.

The human body is magnificent. YOUR body is magnificent! It was created to weigh your ideal weight. This is excellent news! It means that your body already agrees (and wants to) to weigh your ideal weight!

Your mind is pretty impressive too. This is more good news. You see, your mind also knows that your body was created to be your perfect weight and your mind knows that your body functions at its best that way. This means that your mind as well as your body already agrees to weigh your ideal weight. Perfect! At least now we have a starting point.

READ THIS AGAIN

You are responsible for your weight.

Your body is unique and you must tune into your unique self.

Losing weight takes change, determination, knowledge, consistency, and effort.

You already have the tools you need to be successful!

Your body wants to weigh your ideal weight.

THE FOUR KEYS

Without a Key, You Can't Unlock the Puzzle

What puzzle? That wonderful but mysteriously unique body you have that requires its own personal combination to be successful in weight loss and weight maintenance. Your body *is* the puzzle and *you* are the one in charge of putting the pieces together. Your body requires a specific combination of elements working together. It will take investigation. It will take time. It will be a magnificent journey of discovery that will sometimes test your patience…and it will be worth it!

By embracing your own uniqueness, you can truly begin the process of providing yourself with your own personal tools for success. It's time to stop comparing your body to other people. Your body will react to you at its own perfect pace and manner, just like it was designed to.

The Keys

The four essential keys to weight loss are:

🔑 *How you think.*

🔑 *How you eat.*

🔑 *How you move.*

🔑 *How you are.*

These are all critical components to having a healthy body weight. When one is off kilter, it affects the others. In other words, they are all so intertwined and connected to each other that when one of those areas is not where it should be, then the other areas become difficult to manage. This is not to suggest that all areas must be perfect at all times. In fact, if one "key" is strong it can help to balance out a weaker "key" provided it's not for a significant length of time.

It's about creating balance; in this case, a balanced lifestyle. It may help to think of it in the literal sense of the word. Imagine trying to balance four items on a pivot point. If they aren't placed properly, everything will be out of balance. With the issue of body weight, when the key factors are out of balance your body weight will reflect it; whether you are overweight or underweight.

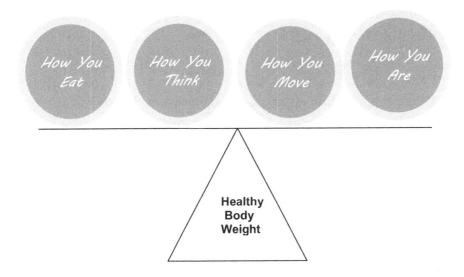

Now before we get too far into this, let's define these areas a bit more (I'll cover it more thoroughly later on, I promise).

"How you eat" means what you eat and drink, how much you eat and drink, and the reasons why you do so.

"How you think" is referring to how you think and feel about yourself, and how you react to those thoughts. It's also referring to your conscious decision making skills, as well as your subconscious habits.

"How you move" means how much you move or exercise your body, in what ways, and how often.

"How you are" refers to any physiological challenges that might need addressing, such as metabolic, genetic, medical, hormonal, or thyroid issues. It also refers to whether or not you actively work towards improving your health.

Every "key" is connected to another one. It has a continuous cycle of cause and effect, so we need to take a closer look at how they link together, because these links explain a lot, including why you might currently be frustrated with weight loss.

This cycle of the keys can be a negative one or a positive one. Negative or broken connections cause and explain weight issues. Positive, balanced, and connected keys lead to your body's ideal and healthiest weight, and a healthier life overall.

By understanding these keys and their connections to each other, you can start identifying which keys you personally may need to fine tune, and importantly really start looking at the big picture. So let's look at these connections and see how they affect each other.

The NEGATIVE Connection between the Keys

Every "key" is connected to another one, no matter which way you look at it. It has a constant domino effect. For example:

>*Key #1 (think) affects key #2 (eat)* because thoughts in the subconscious mind controls your habits. Poor eating habits can cause weight problems.

>*Key #1 (think) affects key #3 (move)* for the same basic reason. The thoughts in the subconscious mind control habits (keep in mind that habits can include physical reactions but also habitual

thought patterns, positive or negative). Poor exercise habits cause weight problems.

Key #1 (think) affects key #4 (are) because a person can believe that they are hostage to physical circumstances. This negative belief system can become a self- fulfilling prophesy.

Key #2 (eat) affects key #1 (think) because the lack of proper nutrition affects the mood center of the brain and your ability to concentrate. Additionally, when we eat foods that we know are not good for us, it usually causes negative emotions such as guilt or depression over our food choice or lack of will power. This can start a whole chain reaction of negative self talk in the mind and affect how we think of ourselves.

Key #2 (eat) affects key #3 (move) because when the body isn't fueled properly it doesn't function as well. This can cause the metabolism to slow and make exercise less effective. It also can make exercise more difficult, uncomfortable, and leave you feeling totally drained after a workout instead of invigorated.

Key #2 (eat) affects key #4 (are) because our food choices directly affect the health of our cells. Food has the ability to heal or create disease, as well as affect weight.

Key #3 (move) affects key #1 (think) because if we don't exercise successfully and get results, then we get discouraged and start thinking negative "I can't do it" types of thoughts which only further causes more failure.

Key #3 (move) affects key #2 (eat) because if we don't balance activity with fuel (food) intake properly, then we can feel ravished after an exercise session and overeat or even feel sick to our stomachs afterwards which can cause us to skip meals which confuses the metabolism and doesn't physically feel very good either.

Key #3 (move) affects key #4 (are) because if we don't understand what our bodies need in terms of exercise in our current state of health, we can cause more strain for the body.

Key #4 (are) affects key #1 (think) because it can create a negative belief system which can negatively impact mood and even create feelings such as hopelessness.

Key #4 (are) affects key #2 (eat) because health conditions can affect food choices and can also contribute to cravings.

Key #4 (are) affects key #3 (move) because it can create a negative "I can't" belief system which can cause people to avoid the exercise that can make them feel better.

Notice how you can take this all a step further. You can add the third and/or forth key into any of the negative puzzle combinations. For example: Key #1 (think) affects key #2 (eat), which then affects key #3 (move) which affects key #4 (are). This applies to all of the combinations, no matter which key you start with.

Many times you encounter a full cycle. For example: Key #1 (think) affects key #2 (eat), which then affects key #3 (move), which affects key #1 (think), which affects key #4 (are)....and so on. Again, this applies no matter what order you start with.

Key #1 (think) seems to bear a lot of collateral damage no matter which negative cycle you encounter. While you can't weigh thoughts on a scale, a person's thoughts can be the heaviest of all. Negative body images can be difficult to overcome and self confidence and self esteem are easily damaged. The negative self-talk can run rampant and become the dominant messages in our minds and change our beliefs in ourselves with the constant bombardment of negative feelings and messages.

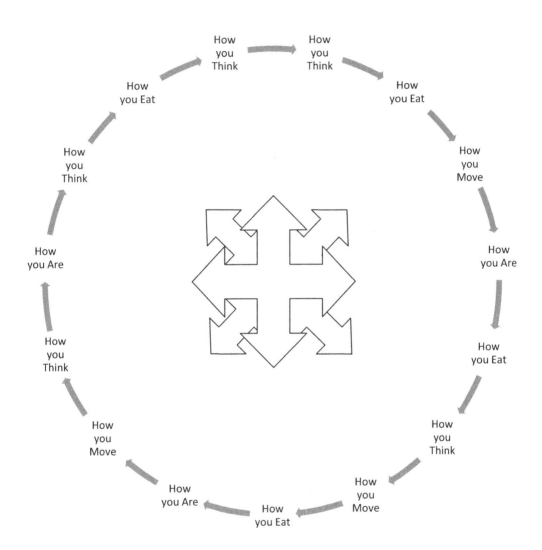

Fortunately, there is a flip side to this. When we create positive connections, we open the door for lifelong change and improved health.

The POSITIVE Connection between the keys

Now let's look at the same cycle from a different perspective. What if the keys could *help* us maintain a healthy weight or lose unwanted weight? Does the connected constant domino effect still apply? Of course! While a broken, neglected or ignored key can cause negative effects on the body, putting <u>all</u> of the keys to work has a positive effect and they still connect and affect one another. For example:

> ***Key #1 (think) affects key #2 (eat)*** because thoughts in the subconscious mind control your habits…good habits included! Appropriate, good eating habits help control weight.

> ***Key #1 (think) affects key #3 (move)*** for the same basic reason. The thoughts in the subconscious mind control habits (keep in mind that habits can include physical reactions but also habitual thought patterns, positive or negative). Positive exercise habits help control body weight.

> ***Key #1 (think) affects key #4 (are)*** because a positive mental state is an empowered one! Attitude and action improves health.

> ***Key #2 (eat) affects key #1 (think)*** because proper nutrition affects the mood center of the brain and assists with your ability to concentrate. Additionally, when we eat foods that we know are good for us, we naturally eliminate negative feelings that are often associated with "the bad foods" or "bad" eating habits. Nobody ever feels guilty, embarrassed, or ashamed of eating their vegetables.

> ***Key #2 (eat) affects key #3 (move)*** because when the body is fueled properly it functions well. Proper nutrition at the correct intervals and amounts assist the metabolism and causes exercise to be more efficient and effective. Eating the right food, in the right amounts, and at the right times also makes exercise easier and prevents post-exercise fatigue.

Key #2 (eat) affects key #4 (are) because good nutrition gives your body the best opportunity to be its healthiest self.

Key #3 (move) affects key #1 (think) because if we exercise successfully and get results, then we stay encouraged and we feel better about our abilities, thus prompting positive thoughts.

Key #3 (move) affects key #2 (eat) because if we balance activity with proper nutrition, then we feel appropriate levels of hunger post-exercise.

Key #3 (move) affects key #4 (are) because proper movement gives your body the best opportunity to be its best, through increased energy, stamina, strength, joint health, reduced pain, amongst many other benefits.

Key #4 (are) affects key #1 (think) because it can create a positive belief system which can positively impact mood and even create good feelings such as self-love, confidence, hope, empowerment, and control.

Key #4 (are) affects key #2 (eat) because food choices can affect health conditions. If you are playing an involved and positive role in your health, then your food choices become common sense, rather than a struggle.

Key #4 (are) affects key #3 (move) because it can create a positive "I can" belief system which can cause people to integrate the daily exercise that can make them feel better, and increase quality of life.

As before, you can take this all a step further or keep the cycle going. You can add the third and/or forth key into any of the positive puzzle combinations. For example: Key #1 (think) affects key #2 (eat), which then affects key #3 (move), which affects key #4 (are). This applies to all of the combinations, no matter which key you start with.

With the keys working in a positive connected state, key #1 (think) seems to get a lot of kudos no matter which positive cycle you encounter. A person's thoughts are powerful and have a major impact on self confidence, self-esteem, and body image. Positive self-talk can be the dominant messages in our minds and encourage our beliefs in ourselves with the constant re-enforcement of positive feelings and messages, thus affecting the actual outcome (us).

So What Does This Mean?

It's all connected. Our thoughts affect our actions. Our actions affect our thoughts. The mind and the body are intimately tangled with each other in such a way that one cannot be affected without causing a reaction to the other. This dynamic holds true to all aspects involving the body, but is particularly obvious with regard to body weight. One cannot begin to effectively achieve weight loss success on a permanent level without taking this into consideration. Certainly, people lose weight all of the time without addressing this big picture view of the mind-body connection, which can also certainly explain why the vast majority of those people will gain back any weight lost at some point or another, and usually end up gaining even more.

The keys are a reflection of this mind-body connection. When one or more of the keys are neglected, over looked, under respected, or underestimated, then physical issues are more likely to rise with regard to body weight or health, whether that is excessive weight issues, underweight issues, eating disorders, or other health problems.

For weight loss to be permanent, all of the issues that can potentially be contributing to the weight issue need to be addressed in a healthy, realistic, and common sense manner. For example, weight loss can be achieved solely through changing nutritional practices, whether they are healthy practices or not. However, it is unlikely that weight loss will be permanent if the other issues are not properly addressed. Of course unhealthy dietary practices should be avoided anyway.

Naturally, this holds true with the other keys as well. A person can exercise for hours a day and still continue to gain weight. A person can learn to think more positively or to use meditation, hypnosis techniques, or other subconscious retraining methods to change habits, but without the proper education on what the body needs to change and an understanding of why those habits need changing, the whole thing can become moot.

Let's face it. There's a lot of misinformation on weight loss and it's caused a lot of confusion and frustration. This is why it's so critical to understand the body from an honest and functional perspective. A person can make tremendous effort in exercising or changing dietary habits, but if those changes aren't actually correct for their body, then it is all a waste.

People are constantly bomb-barded with food and diet information and a good portion of it is inaccurate. It's no wonder that people are confused! The lesson here? Cover the bases and assume nothing. Nearly every dieter I have ever met has told me that they "know what foods to eat but they just don't do it." Upon exploration of their dietary habits I find that only about 2% of them are accurate with that statement. What it really takes is a deeper understanding of how the body actually *functions* on certain foods, which we'll explore more later. The same can be said regarding exercise. A person can spend hours and hours at the gym and get nowhere. Your body has its own combination of what works. Get the combination wrong, and you won't likely be satisfied with the results. You have to tune into your body. Work with it. Understand it. Love it. Be honest. Tune out the garbage. Tune into the truth and you will be okay.

Understand the keys. Analyze and process them all.

READ THIS AGAIN

The keys to weight loss are:

☞ *How you think.*

☞ *How you eat.*

☞ *How you move.*

☞ *How you are.*

When the key factors are out of balance your body weight will reflect it.

Every "key" affects the other keys, no matter how you look at it.

When one or more of the keys are neglected, weight issues are likely.

A person's thoughts are powerful and have a major impact on self confidence, self-esteem, and body image.

Our thoughts affect our actions. Our actions affect our thoughts.

The mind and the body are tangled with each other in such a way that one cannot be affected without causing a reaction to the other.

You have to tune into your body. Work with it. Understand it. Love it. Be honest. Tune out the garbage. Tune into the truth and you will be okay.

CHAPTER 4

HOW THOUGHTS CREATE OUR BODIES

Here is where we begin to explore key #1 (how you think) and its connection to body weight. The truth is that our thoughts are powerful and they can create our reality, which of course affects our body. This all gets pretty deep so it's best to start at the beginning rather than jumping head first into the mind-body connection and the science of neurobiology.

Whether you want to call it self-talk, the law of attraction, self-fulfilling prophecy, meditation, affirmations, hypnosis, self-hypnosis, sub-consciousness, visualization, or whatever title you feel the most comfortable with, it all breaks down to the same thing; Our thoughts, what we do with them, and how they affect us.

What we think can become what we believe, which becomes who we are and how we react to our world, as well as how we treat ourselves and others. Thus our thoughts create our experience in the world, good or bad. What many people assume is that we just mosey along in this world in some sort of pre-determined fate and we just get bounced around from situation to situation according to that destiny…sort of like being the pinball in a giant pinball machine.

The reality is that we have the ability to change our path because we can always choose our reaction and our action. The problem is that most people aren't taught this truth, leaving many to feel helpless, become victims, or to feel like they are trapped or enslaved by their own habits or fears. Also, there is conscious thought and action, as well as subconscious thought and actions. Even though the brain belongs to the same person, the conscious and subconscious mind might be on two totally different paths, which is why we need to more deeply understand how our brain organizes and uses information so that we can control it better.

So why do we need to spend time understanding the differences between our conscious and our subconscious mind? Because, your subconscious mind is dominant. <u>Your subconscious mind controls your habits</u>, which means it's ultimately controlling exercise habits, eating habits, and self-talk/thinking habits. It's even playing a role in our ability to combat and overcome physical issues and disease. Obviously, proper and healthy habits and behaviors create healthier bodies! With that in mind, it's probably a good idea that we get to understand how our brain works a little better.

Conscious Thinking VS Subconscious Thinking

We use different parts of our brain for different things. For example, the conscious mind is used when a person is very focused on a project or actively engaged in learning something new, but actually plays a smaller role in our everyday life and in who we are and how we behave. The subconscious mind is dominant, and plays the biggest role into who we are and who we become, however it's not a logic based mind. Emotions, habits, learned behaviors and responses are part of the subconscious brain. Additionally, our conscious mind processes far less information, far slower that our subconscious mind. The exact numbers are debatable, but many experts agree that we are only using our conscious brain about 10% of the time, which means the subconscious brain (the other 90%), is the true powerhouse.

Since the subconscious mind is such a dominant factor in our lives (and our body weight), it stands to reason that we want to be able to learn how to understand and control this better, or at least learn how to favorably work with it in order to get better outcomes.

Our minds operate on a conscious and a subconscious level simultaneously. Most people are under the impression that they are going about their day-to-day business using their conscious brain/mind as they go about their activities, when in actuality they are hardly using their conscious mind at all in comparison to the subconscious or unconscious mind. Our habits and patterns are controlled by the subconscious mind, even when they are habits we prefer we didn't have. Often times we intend on doing one thing (consciously), but we end up doing something else (subconscious behavior takes over). For example, when a person intends to eat healthy, but can't seem to resist the urge to eat junk. We think it's about will power, when it's actually a power struggle between our conscious and subconscious mind. In other words, there's a battle going on in the mind. Once we begin to understand that, it all starts becoming more obvious that it should actually be about knowing how to redirect our mind in a more productive way, so we can quiet the internal battle. And yes, there's a way to do that.

THE MIND'S OPERATING SYSTEMS:
Conscious, Subconscious, and Unconscious Thinking

The terms "subconscious" and "unconscious" are often used interchangeably when actually they are two distinct and different categories within the mind's operating systems. In fact, not only should it rightly be defined under three operating systems (as opposed to two), but those operating systems can be affected by one another. Additionally, actions, thoughts, activities, and bodily functions can come from more than one operating system simultaneously. This will become important as we start understanding the role of brain activity in regards to weight loss.

The Conscious Mind
The conscious mind is used for higher thinking processes, as when a person is very focused on a project or actively engaged in learning something new, when the mind is very connected to the activity and repetitive familiarity has not yet taken place. For example, when a person is learning a new dance move, the conscious mind is the dominant brain. But as we practice that dance move, the subconscious mind gradually becomes the dominant brain. In other words, once we've mastered a given activity, the brain changes the operating system in which in uses. As things become thoughts that we *know*, it switches over to the subconscious operating system, where

the data is stored and can easily be brought up (whether we want it to or not).

Another example of this learning transfer from the conscious brain to the subconscious brain is putting on our clothes. When you were a child, it was once difficult to put on your clothes and manage zippers and buttons. Your conscious brain was very busy in this phase! I bet that today when you got dressed the mechanics of *how* to zip a zipper or button a button was a "no-brainer" for you. Actually…it wasn't a "no-brainer", but it's so easy for you now that it's a *subconscious* activity. You've experienced this dominant brain shifting with thousands of things. Eventually, the subconscious takes over (nearly always).

The Unconscious Mind

Your unconscious mind controls basic functions such as breathing, digestion, circulation, perspiration, balance, coordination, and the release of hormones. In other words, the unconscious mind/brain controls things that happen automatically in order to allow the body to function.

Our conscious brain can interact with the unconscious brain to some extent. This means that while we can consciously choose to blink, the conscious mind can't entirely take over that process. We are not able to consciously decide to just stop blinking for the rest of our waking hours. Our unconscious mind will eventually cause us to blink, no matter what the conscious mind attempts to do. The same can be said of other unconscious activities such as breathing. Sure, you can consciously take deep or shallow breaths or change the tempo of your breathing, or even hold your breath for a couple of minutes. However, as long as you are alive, your unconscious mind will force you to breath. So while there's a small modicum of control by the conscious mind, ultimately, this is the domain of the unconscious mind and the unconscious mind is the dominant operating system of these areas.

Some categorize the subconscious and unconscious brain together, but they are ultimately separate. The reason being is that we can "re-train" our subconscious to react differently, but we can't "re-train" our unconscious brain to over-ride automatic bodily function. We can't train our unconscious brain to start pumping our blood backwards. Basically, the unconscious is on auto-pilot, which is a good thing. We are busy enough working with the other parts of the brain.

The Subconscious Mind

The subconscious mind is an incredible part of us and a dominant factor in the make up of whom we are, however it's not necessarily a logic based mind. It does not think in linear terms. Instead it is a parallel processor. Emotions, habits, belief systems, learned behaviors and responses are part of this operating system.

The general train of thought is that the subconscious mind is the culprit in all mental disorders. Generally with mental disorders, the thinking is involuntary and not under control. Thoughts can be overcrowded and confusing. It's difficult to hide or control bad thoughts, and those thoughts can be converted into actions more easily. Chemical imbalances aside, these are all traits of the subconscious operating system of the mind.

This is not to suggest that the subconscious mind is a bad thing, but rather to point out that it's very powerful because it controls our responses, reactions, habits, thought processes and behaviors in such a way that it defines who we are. Think about this; when someone describes your personality they will usually use adjectives that are descriptors of the behaviors that are driven by the subconscious mind. If a person is defined as being a "real jerk" it's because that person repeatedly displays *behaviors* that are perceived that way. Those behaviors are actually habitual responses which were learned for one reason or another at sometime by the conscious mind but at some point transitioned into subconscious *behavior* which then manifested itself in actions and reactions and thus became a part of who that "jerk" is!

Since logic doesn't necessarily prevail in this huge operating system of a subconscious brain, we can find ourselves thinking useless, unproductive, and untrue thoughts which our conscious mind disagrees with from a logical perspective and we can find ourselves in a battle of rationality and will power, while often losing that battle. Ultimately, the subconscious nearly always wins.

For example, a person who has suffered sexual abuse may find it difficult to enjoy a healthy sex life in marriage. Logically, the conscious mind knows that their consensual partner is not the same person who hurt them and doesn't have any intention of hurting them. However, the subconscious mind still has a negative association to sex and still retains emotional control, thus prohibiting or interfering with the enjoyment of sex with a loving partner.

Another example is the person who is trying to lose weight and they know (consciously) that they don't want or need to eat cookies yet they don't have the willpower so they eat them anyway (subconscious activity).

Conscious brain activity can influence subconscious brain activity, but this is often for short term decision making and in the case of weight loss, can be a struggle. For example, a person at a buffet might intend on choosing salad (conscious choice), but ends up with a plate full of fried foods (the dominate subconscious mind overpowered the conscious mind's initial decision).

Naturally, the best solution is to consciously address and reprogram or redirect the subconscious mind in a way that is beneficial, and actually helps you reach your goals. To get there, we still need to understand more about how the subconscious mind computes input. More importantly, how to change it.

READ THIS AGAIN

What we think can become what we believe, which becomes who we are and how we react to our world, as well as how we treat ourselves and others.

The reality is that we have the ability to change our path because we can always choose our reaction and our action.

Your subconscious mind controls your habits, which means it's ultimately controlling exercise habits, eating habits, and self-talk/thinking habits.

Many experts agree that we are only using our conscious brain about 10% of the time, which means the subconscious brain (the other 90%), is the true powerhouse.

CHAPTER 5

THE POWER OF SELF-TALK

The words that are floating around in your head are thoughts, and thoughts are powerful. Self-talk, whether supportive or critical has the power to change and create beliefs, which then alters perceptions and outcomes. In other words, self-talk matters, perhaps more than you think.

Negative self-talk generates more negativity, which is usually not a person's deliberate goal. For most people the goal is to *reduce* negativity. In order to reduce it, we have to stop or re-direct negative self-talk. The challenge is that it's not always as straight forward as it seems to do that.

One of the factors that can prevent the positive self-talk from taking root in our minds is that the conscious mind and the subconscious mind can work together simultaneously or entirely independently from each other. They (the conscious and subconscious) can hear the same exact words either from an outside source or through our self-talk and potentially have opposite reactions! For example, the conscious mind hears all words and prefers the grammar that feels comfortable to you. Conversely, grammar is relatively irrelevant to the subconscious mind and the subconscious mind only hears select words and completely ignores other words. As it turns out, this is actually a big deal, because even when we are trying to be more positive or change habits through self-talk, the approach could be rendered completely ineffective according to how the subconscious mind interpreted the thought.

Here is a prime example of that dynamic: The subconscious mind doesn't register negative modifiers in language, depending on where they are placed in a sentence. In other words, it doesn't hear words such as "no", "don't", or "not." This means that we can accidentally reinforce the very thought we didn't want!

For example: We say....

"No more fast food."
Our subconscious hears: *"~~No~~ more fast food".*

"Don't be nervous."
Our subconscious hears: *"~~Don't~~ be nervous."*

"I'm not going to eat the cookies."
Our subconscious hears: *"I'm ~~not~~ going to eat the cookies."*

"I don't want to keep procrastinating"
Our subconscious mind hears *"I ~~don't~~ want to keep procrastinating."*

Do you See the problem that this presents?

Basically, every time you say or think a statement with a negative modifier in it, you are embedding the subconscious mind with the exact opposite of what you wanted! In essence, you are programming your subconscious mind to work against you!

Remember, the subconscious mind is a *powerhouse*, controlling up to *90%* of the outcome, including habits, perceptions, and behaviors. So if we are using the "don't", "not", and "no" words we could actually be making this harder for ourselves!

Let's compound the issue by the fact that we create images or pictures in our minds when we speak or think, which further demonstrates the point that our subconscious mind doesn't process the negatives as we would wish it would.

Let's try this out. I'm going to ask you to simply *not* do something. Ready to not do it? Okay, here goes.
- Do *not* think about what a stop sign looks like.
- Definitely *don't* think about what color the stop sign is.
- *Or how about...* Don't think about the size or shape of an elephant.

How did it go?

I'm guessing that you know what a red stop sign looks like and you know what an elephant is. Therefore, then when I mentioned the name of the object (stop sign or elephant), your mind conjured up the image in your head, even though I asked you *not* to. Why? Because the subconscious mind does not compute the negative modifiers in language, it focuses on the *subject*. Grammar and proper English are irrelevant. You are dealing with an emotional brain that computes with images, memories, and sensory input.

Now consider the issue when it comes to losing weight. What happens when someone says *"I'm not going to eat those donuts"*? That is the ultimate double whammy set-up for the subconscious mind. Not only does it hear *"I'm going to eat those donuts"*, but it also gets an image of the donuts! Sometimes even a mental image of the person eating the donuts and even a memory of what the donuts taste like and that the donuts taste good. So given all of this, perhaps it is better understood why people "give in" to the donuts or why they "couldn't quit thinking about the donuts" or seem to have a lack of "willpower". In fact, just reading this paragraph involving donuts will spark some readers to start craving donuts. Interesting, isn't it?

This subconscious brain quirk is important to remember. It can make the difference as to whether or not you are making things harder or easier on yourself.

Our high level minds still function on a primitive scale, no matter how intellectual we like to think we are. Book smarts cannot override the primitive nature of certain mental, emotional, and physical responses, which includes how the subconscious filters (or doesn't filter) information and messages.

Using Self-talk to Your Advantage
An easy way to avoid adding difficulty is by focusing on what we *want*, rather than what we *don't want*. In order to get the right image and message in your subconscious mind, learn to say what you *want*. When we

do that, we get more of our intended outcome because the subconscious mind actually receives the intended message. The words that we use to describe the situation in our minds and in our spoken words make a huge difference in what our outcome becomes.

Does it work instantly and perfectly? Not always. Like many things, it takes practice. But with repetition, the new self-talk changes into a new pattern of thinking.

"I don't want to eat junk food anymore" and "I want to stop eating junk food" may sound like the same thing to your conscious mind, but they are opposites in the subconscious mind. So the real problem becomes that we are potentially making it much harder on ourselves by not choosing language that directs our subconscious mind towards our goals. If we focus on what we don't want, we are actually *reinforcing* what we don't want and making things much harder than it needs to be.

Think of it this way…when you order in a restaurant you tell the waiter what you want. Right? You may be thinking that you want a bowl of soup, but the waiter can't conclude that you want a bowl of soup just because you say *"I don't want a hamburger."* The only way to make it clear to the waiter what it is that you want to order is by telling the waiter what you *do* want, not what you *don't* want. Our subconscious mind works the same way. We must learn to speak to it in terms of what we *do* want, rather than what we *don't* want.

Here are examples of *focusing on what we want*:

Instead of *"No more fast food"*, try *"I'm avoiding fast food."*
Our subconscious hears: *"I'm avoiding fast food."*

Instead of *"Don't be nervous"*, try *"I am calm."*
Our subconscious hears: *"I am calm."*

31

Instead of *"I'm not going to eat the cookies"*, try *"Cookies make me feel sluggish"* or *"I am eating foods that create health"* or *"I am ignoring the cookies."*

Our subconscious hears: *"Cookies make me feel sluggish"* or *"I am eating foods that create health"* or *"I am ignoring the cookies."*

Instead of *"I don't want to keep procrastinating"*, try *"I am going to get started right now."*

Our subconscious mind hears *"I am going to get started right now."*

Now the subconscious is hearing the *intended* message, and can start creating new belief patterns that you actually want.

There's a catch.

What if you don't *believe* the new words? Let's take this thought: "Don't be nervous". You can re-direct your self-talk to what you do want by saying "I am calm", and it can work <u>IF</u> it's believable to you. If you are a nervous wreck and mentally repeating the words "I am calm" feel ridiculous to you, then the subconscious mind won't *believe* "I am calm" and won't change the course. In that case, sometimes we have to take baby steps, and gradually work our thoughts towards our desired outcome. So if "I am calm" doesn't feel *believable,* maybe something like "I have the *ability* to be calm" feels more realistic and is therefore more effective. Once you can mentally get yourself from "Nervous" to "I have the ability to be calm", it then becomes easier to continue the transition to feeling calmer. Perhaps the next mental step would be "I am *becoming* calmer." Other words might help this as well…supportive words that reinforce the outcome, such as "I am confident" or "I am safe" or "I am okay."

Fair warning… this takes a little practice, especially if you were in the habit of negative self-talk, but the practice of re-directing self-talk is a very useful tool and can ultimately change outcomes and eliminate unwanted thoughts and habits.

The lesson here is: Listen to your self-talk. If it's supportive and phrased towards the desired outcome then give yourself a mental high-five! If it's negative or focused on what you don't want, take the time to re-direct the thought. You have the power to create new pathways, new outcomes, and new opportunities. This helps you change your body and your health. Your thoughts are powerful. Choose wisely.

Using Positive Affirmations

There is an obvious benefit to learning how to think of things in your mind using positive (what you _do_ want) verbiage as opposed to negative (what you _don't_ want) verbiage both in the form of auditory expression and in our mental thoughts.

The words and messages that replay themselves in one's mind can become embedded in one's subconscious, thus affecting behaviors, beliefs, and forming habits. This is a very powerful phenomenon that impacts outcome and has a tremendous impact on a person's life. It then becomes clearer as to why learning to master this is so important.

The words we repeat in our minds are a form of self-programming and you can consciously and deliberately choose to alter the outcome by controlling or maneuvering the messages that are allowed to run through the mind. This takes practice, time, and effort and can be quite challenging for people to do on a consistent basis. However, with practice, it's a skill that can be mastered.

Positive affirmations are a piece of this process. Having a few positive mantras can really help to get past a struggle point. Some people benefit by having a few "go-to" mantras to over-rule commonly occurring negative self-talk, especially if they are not skilled at quickly re-framing. However, we must be realistic about the process and realize that perfection isn't the goal because life isn't perfect. Life still happens, along with the ups and downs that accommodate it. It's just that people who have a more positive

33

mindset, tend to do better, even when life throws some tough curveballs, which is another reason to put this skill to good use.

The path to weight loss isn't a straight and easy one. There will be curves, mountains, and even some back-slides. But if we keep our head in the game and working for us, we will get to where we wanted to be.

The only person you can truly control is you.

When one learns to master the majority of their thoughts and change their subconscious thinking patterns, one still has to understand that the only person that changed was themselves. Now there is still a net reaction, because as you change yourself, it changes how other people perceive you and alters how they respond to you.

You've no doubt heard the expression "Your perception is your reality." That's because your perception and your *projection* creates your reality. You can ultimately only control your own thoughts and reactions. This is great news that you can't control other people because then that would mean that they can control you, which would be disastrous! You have the ability to control your own perceptions which then has a trickle effect on other people and how they interact with you which changes your experience in the world.

So why bother mastering having a positive attitude and practicing positive affirmations? Because they are an important form of re-training the subconscious mind.

Our self talk plays a vital role in our beliefs, our behaviors, and our outcome. The trick is to practice positive self-talk and positive affirmations enough so that the practice of positive thinking becomes a habit as well.

So by now we already know that negative self-talk or using negative verbiage doesn't provide us with a positive outcome. However, if we focus on what we want rather than what we don't want, our odds greatly improve for having a positive outcome. Some refer to this process as reframing.

34

Reframing

Reframing is a technique that causes a shift in attitude and responsibility. This method of communicating can come from your own internal communication or come from an external source.

Recently I was watching the television show about people working with personal trainers to lose weight. I decided to listen closely to how the individual trainers were speaking to the people they were training. I noticed that some people were deeply attached to their trainer and other people were obviously disconnected from their trainer. The trainer that had established rapport was very skilled in the art of reframing and speaking with positive verbiage, even when he was being "tough" on them. He was very skilled at embedding positive imagery in the minds of his clients thus causing them to feel very connected and motivated in spite of the challenges and physical demands.

The other trainer on the show was not skilled in reframing or positive messaging, and it also clearly showed. Her clients were experiencing a disconnect and having to struggle just as much with the emotional challenges of exercise as they were the physical challenges of exercise. Basically, the experience was miserable for them.

Reframing has to do with shifting perspectives. Often people get in the habit of being very negative and expect failure even when they think they are *trying* to succeed. No wonder it's so difficult!

Recognizing negative self-talk is the first step towards shifting your attitude. Taking personal responsibility for your situation and your circumstances is another important step.

If your perceptions become your reality then it is a very good idea to gain some positive perceptions!

Bad Things Still Happen

So with all of this positivity floating around now everything should be perfect, right? Not the last time I checked. Life still has normal ups and downs. Tragedies still occur. Accidents still happen. Other people's decisions, reactions, and behaviors still have an effect on us. We can't control other people. We can only control ourselves. We can only control our own reaction to things. Bad things still happen to people who practice positive thinking, that's inevitable. The difference is that a person who practices positive thinking tends to recover from a bad situation much quicker and suffers less physical stress and symptoms. Simply put, they cope better.

Can You Do It Alone?

It's certainly possible to change your subconscious thoughts by making a conscious decision to learn how to positively self-talk, reframe, and redirect the messages that come into your mind. It's also absolutely possible to do this all on your own. However for some people the skills simply don't come naturally and there is such a habit of background self-sabotage that they simply cannot fully grasp these concepts deeply enough or practice them long enough in order for them to make an effective change.

Sometimes a person is often better off by employing the help of a trained and qualified hypnotherapist or cognitive psychotherapist to help them make changes with their subconscious thoughts. A properly trained therapist should possess the language skills to properly motivate the subconscious mind to change.

With or without help, it takes practice and that's okay. Just remember that you are worth the time it takes to practice working with your mind in this way. Your mind is part of the weight loss puzzle. Taking the time to learn how to better control and work with your own mind will be a tremendous benefit, and make the weight loss journey not only easier, but actually enjoyable.

Changing Thoughts with Some Help

There are several ways to change thinking patterns, whether you change them yourself or enlist the help of a qualified therapist (preferably one that specializes in weight loss and subconscious thinking).

One of the most direct paths to change the subconscious mind is through hypnotherapy, whether you are assisted by a professional, use recordings, or use self-hypnosis techniques. The American Medical Association has classified hypnosis as a treatment tool since the 1950s.

Unfortunately, hypnosis is often greatly misunderstood and is plagued with myths and misconceptions, which causes apprehension and misunderstanding. Certainly movies, books, internet fallacies, and stage show performers have added to the confusion. Additionally, finding a properly trained and experienced therapist can be tricky, as the profession is completely unregulated in most states. This means that as a consumer, you will need to do your homework to ensure that your "hypnotherapist" is properly educated and experienced. Once you find qualified help, hypnosis can be an excellent tool provided you understand the process.

There's nothing mysterious about hypnosis at all, in spite of what the movies or stage show performers would like you to believe. It's simply a way of working with how we think. There's no such thing as mind control and nobody can make you do anything you don't want to do. Your morals, ethics, and values cannot be altered in hypnosis, nor can someone take control of you in any way. It is not a passive process. In fact, in order for it to work, it must be about what *you* want. Hypnosis will not work for someone who doesn't really want to change. Hypnosis isn't about losing control or relinquishing control at all. It's about *you* having more personal control. True hypnotherapy professionals know this and are willing to explain it to you.

It's totally safe and is something that the mind naturally already does. In fact, everyone actually goes in and out of hypnosis all day long without even being aware of it.

Have you ever missed an exit while driving? That's actually called "highway hypnosis." It's an example of how our brain will switch from a conscious activity to a subconscious activity. In the example of highway hypnosis, you started out driving with BOTH sides of your brain, but at some point your conscious mind wandered off and started thinking about other things, so your subconscious brain took over the act of driving the vehicle. By the time you noticed it with your conscious brain, you had already missed your exit.

On average, almost 2½ times as much weight is lost by incorporating hypnosis compared to those people not using hypnosis. Why? Because it takes into account your subconscious thinking patterns and helps you to re-direct them. Hypnosis facilitates weight loss by making the change from bad habits to good habits easier. That's it! It's not mysterious at all actually. The key is that one needs to know which specific habits need changing *before* starting any kind of hypnosis (self hypnosis or with the help of a professional).

There are also common pleasant side effects with the use of hypnosis. For example, a person seeking help with weight loss by using hypnosis may discover that their self-esteem, self-confidence, and self worth are improving in addition to undergoing the process of losing weight. It's simply because the subconscious mind is wise to what is truly needed for the individual and will "listen" to what the person really needs, even if the person doesn't consciously recognize what those needs really are.

It's an interesting phenomenon as well as a highly beneficial one. It stems from the fact that we have a body and mind that understands the need for self preservation. So even when we may not recognize what is truly lacking in terms of our sense of self satisfaction, contentment, and happiness, our subconscious mind clearly understands what is needed.

READ THIS AGAIN

Self-talk, whether supportive or critical has the power to change and create beliefs.

They (the conscious and subconscious) can hear the same exact words either from an outside source or through our self-talk and potentially have opposite reactions!

The subconscious mind is a powerhouse, controlling up to 90% of the outcome, including habits, perceptions, and behaviors.

The subconscious mind doesn't register negative modifiers in language, depending on where they are placed in a sentence.

In order to get the right image and message in your subconscious mind, learn to say what you want.

The path to weight loss isn't a straight and easy one. There will be curves, mountains, and even some back-slides. But if we keep our head in the game and working for us, we will get to where we wanted to be.

The words and messages that replay themselves in one's mind can become embedded in one's subconscious, thus affecting behaviors, beliefs, and forming habits.

Listen to your self-talk. Reframe it if needed.

You have the power to create new pathways, new outcomes, and new opportunities.

If your perceptions become your reality then it is a good idea to gain some positive perceptions!

Your perception and your projection create your reality.

Your thoughts are powerful. Choose wisely.

CHAPTER 6

SELF-FULLFILLING PROPHACY

You've met those people...the ones who constantly complain. They complain about their bad relationships because they always seem to find themselves in a bad relationship. They complain about their health, and sure enough, they always seem to have something wrong with them. They complain about being broke because they are always poor. They complain about not being about to stop smoking because they always smoke. They complain about being unlucky because luck always eludes them. They complain about not being able to lose weight because they are fat. They will even complain about never finding a parking place, always being stopped at red lights, finding it nearly impossible to make left turns across traffic, always getting behind a bad driver, always having reservations messed up, and on and on and on, and it's likely that they are right! They will "wake up on the wrong side of the bed" and be crabby all day. They will be "exhausted" and be miserably tired and barely able to function. If they are "depressed", they are. If they "could never accomplish *that*", they won't. Pretty simple actually.

Henry Ford was quoted as saying, "Whether you think you can or think you can't, you are usually right." I agree with Henry. While it may not be an absolute, the majority of the time you are the creator of your personal destiny, your experiences, your interactions with the world, and your outcome. It's your own personal belief system that is generating results, whether you realize it or not. You are participating in your life with your subconscious mind that is producing behaviors even when and if you think you are consciously intending to do something else!

Your subconscious mind directs most of your activities and causes you to behave in certain ways that puts you in certain situations and thus creates the outcome. In other words, *you* are the generator of your own self-fulfilling prophecy! So if you *believe* that you always get stuck in the slowest check-out line in the store, even if you consciously try to pick the fastest line, your subconscious mind actually makes the decision of which line you end up standing in and it becomes more likely that you will end up in a slow line again, thus reaffirming the belief that you always get stuck in the slowest check-out line in the store…because most of the time, you do! This self-fulfilling prophecy manifests itself in all areas of life, even areas that might be more or less obvious.

I know someone who has always been in bad relationships. She always chooses men who are neglectful in one form or another. Even though she can rationalize and recognize the negative traits of these men and consciously proclaim her desire for a "nice guy", she continues to subconsciously choose neglectful men while rejecting men who treat her kindly. So even while consciously she craves kindness, her own (subconscious) belief system prohibits her from being in a healthy relationship.

Self-fulfilling Prophecy and Weight Loss

Let's apply this principle to weight loss. I meet people who come in with a belief already in place with regards to their ability to lose weight. Sometimes it's in the form of an excuse, as when someone tells me that it's their "genetics" that makes them fat. *(That's not true by the way. Body types can be genetic. Obesity is not genetic. Where and how you store fat on your body is genetic. Having too much storage fat is not genetic. Families are collectively fat because they share bad habits, not bad genes.)* Now that that's cleared up, let's go back to examining the connection between a self-fulfilling prophecy and weight loss.

Fat Attitude (beliefs that make you fat)

"I can't lose weight because_____."

"I tried before but_____."

"I want to lose weight but_____."

"That doesn't work for me because_____."

"I would lose weight but_____."

"I don't have time to take care of myself because _____."

No matter what you fill in the blank with, the outcome will be the same. Whether the statement has any real validity or whether it's complete and total nonsense, the outcome will be the same! So whether someone says that "I can't lose weight because I eat 5 candy bars every day" or they say "I can't lose weight because the sky isn't green" they will have the same result! There is no doubt that certain behaviors (like 5 candy bars a day) will cause weight issues and others (like a green sky) will not cause weight issues, however it's the limiting belief that drives behaviors that determine outcome.

When someone tells me they tried exercising before and it didn't work. I know that what *really* happened was that they exercised ineffectively in the past, therefore the ineffective experience formed a belief that exercise doesn't work. I don't believe for one second that exercise doesn't work. That person just didn't know *what* to do or *how* to do it. Until they change their belief system about exercise they won't exercise correctly, even if they have the correct exercise recommendations. *You have to push a mental re-set button on some things in order to even create the possibility of a different outcome.*

You are what you think. Your body does not want or need you to be overweight, so it's not your body that is doing it. It starts in your head. If you believe that you crave sugar or chocolate, or chips, you will! If you think you eat due to emotions, you will! If you think exercise won't work, it won't! If you think you don't have time to exercise or eat right, you won't! Are you seeing a pattern?

Your thoughts determine your outcomes because they cause your behaviors. That means if you believe that you crave sugar then every time you see a sweet or even think of a sweet then you will want the sugary item and you will most likely seek out and eat something sugary, even if you don't want to or didn't intend to. This starts the cycle all over again because it reinforces the belief which then reinforces the behavior. When the behavior is repeated it confirms the belief, and so on.

Belief Systems

People define themselves by their beliefs. If you were to ask someone to honestly define and describe themselves, you would get a laundry list of adjectives that are based on their belief or perception of themselves regardless of whether or not it is actually true or whether or not it is a positive belief or a negative belief. For example, someone may believe themselves to be stupid when they are actually very smart or someone may think that they are gorgeous when actually they are not very attractive at all. Interestingly, the person's belief of themselves creates a pattern of behavior that confirms the belief (to them) and creates a cycle that is repeated until something disrupts that cycle, which may or may not ever occur.

Origin of Belief Systems

Belief systems start in a variety of ways at any age, although children are particularly susceptible to outside influences. Messages that are told to us become part of our belief system unless they are so ridiculous that our minds reject the message. However, children are more easily influenced because they tend to be more open-minded and have yet to form mental barriers grounded in reality. For example, someone may tell an adult that they have a big nose. The adult can then rationally decide whether that message is true. If the adult actually has a normal sized or small nose, then the insult is rejected and does not affect that person's belief system about their nose (although it may affect their belief system with regards to the person who delivered the insult). The same message to a child can have dramatic affects. If a child is told they have a big nose, there's a much higher chance that the statement will become part of the child's belief system even if the child has a normal sized or small nose. The child will much more likely grow up to be self conscious about the size of their nose and may even seek out plastic surgery once they are old enough to pursue such "solutions".

This dynamic is compounded when a message is repeated. If a child is repeatedly told they are worthless or unlovable, they will much more likely to grow up having self-worth and relationship issues that can continue throughout their entire lives. If a child is told they are fat (true or not), they are much more likely to struggle with weight or body image issues as adults.

Message Embedding

Repeating messages can become embedded in the subconscious mind and thus form belief systems which affect our behaviors which produce our outcome or our life experience. For a message to be embedded it has usually been heard a lot. What is surprising to people is that the repetition doesn't always come from an outside source. In fact, the opposite is likely the case.

Obviously, if we hear a message repetitively from an outside source or sources it can be influential. If we are constantly being told we are good at something in particular, then it's likely we are good at it and our belief system continues the cycle of being good at it. The same is true for negative messages. However, we don't need external sources to get that repetitive messaging because our minds will replay messages over and over, particularly if the message was attached to an emotion. Even if something is told to us only once we often repeat that message to ourselves enough to embed that message into part of our belief system. Our belief system determines our responses which then affects our outcome. This means that someone can be given a message one time and our mind will replay that message over and over, so now that person has actually *experienced* that message multiple, hundreds, or even thousands of times. Those are the kinds of messages that *embed* in the subconscious and form our opinions about ourselves and our abilities, both positive and negative, both wanted and unwanted. What's more, even we can logically and consciously recognize that a message is invalid, once it's embedded into the subconscious mind, the message still drives attitude, perceptions, and behavior.

An example of this might be a skinny girl who was told by someone that she is fat. Even though the message is untrue, that message may be played over and over again in that girl's mind, particularly if it evoked an emotional response. As the girl replays that message in her own mind over and over again, she can begin to believe it and begin responding to that negative messaging. This is often what happens in the case of anorexics. People affected by anorexia are often absolutely convinced that they're fat, even though they can be severely underweight. Their perception is their reality and their perception was created by a message that was allowed to replay itself over and over again in the mind.

This unintentional embedded messaging plays a big role in creating our belief system which then creates our habits and can leave us with unwanted and undesirable habits. Part of what becomes necessary is to recognize what those negative messages are and then apply the same principles of repetition to messages that are positive and productive.

Effective positive repetition can significantly change outlook, beliefs, perceptions, response, and outcome. This makes the whole process of creating change much simpler and easier for the individual to undergo and often leads to other pleasant and positive outcomes besides changing the original habit or thought process.

Limiting Belief Systems

Unfortunately, belief systems, whether they have any actual validity or not, can seriously limit a person's potential and have negative consequences on a person's life and ultimately affect their happiness. In most cases, if someone is convinced they can't do something then they won't even try, and even if they do try they tend to give up easily or never take the steps that are necessary to accomplish the goal. They become their own obstacles.

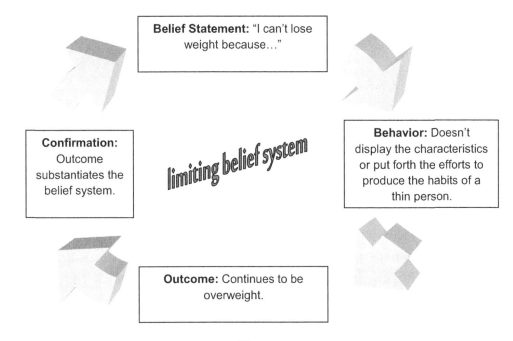

Belief Statement: "I can't lose weight because..."

Behavior: Doesn't display the characteristics or put forth the efforts to produce the habits of a thin person.

Outcome: Continues to be overweight.

Confirmation: Outcome substantiates the belief system.

limiting belief system

Limitless Belief Systems

Fortunately, there are opposites to nearly everything. If there is a negative there can be a positive. If there is a "fat attitude" there can be a "thin attitude". In other words, there is no reason to be trapped by a limiting belief system. Once a person is willing to let go of the excuses and the old mindset, possibility opens up. As a person is willing to recognize the need for change and act in a proactive manner, they unlock the limits.

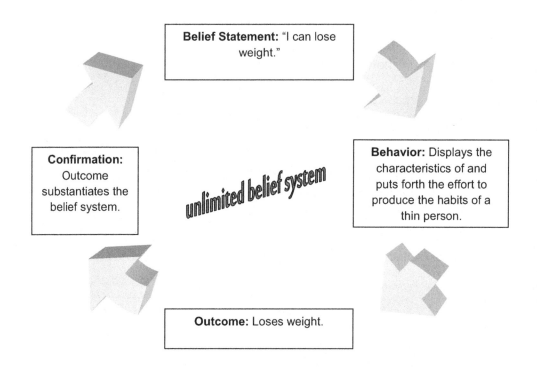

Belief Statement: "I can lose weight."

Behavior: Displays the characteristics of and puts forth the effort to produce the habits of a thin person.

unlimited belief system

Confirmation: Outcome substantiates the belief system.

Outcome: Loses weight.

Let's look at it this way:

Limiting Belief System in Action

If a person with a limiting belief system thinks they will always be fat, then they will fail to prepare themselves to be thin and their subconscious actions will perpetuate a cycle of being overweight which confirms the belief of always being fat.

Unlimited Belief System in Action

If a person with an unlimited belief system who is fat believes they have the real potential to be thin, they will take action to be thin and their subconscious actions will create and support behaviors that facilitate a change in weight.

By changing any limiting belief systems, it produces changes in behavior, attitudes, and reactions that create the opportunity for the goal you desire.

"Luck is what happens when preparation meets opportunity."
Seneca, Roman dramatist, philosopher, & politician (5 BC – 65 AD)

"Success is where preparation and opportunity meet."
Bobby Unser, American car racer who won the Indianapolis 500 race three times

"All our dreams can come true – if we have the courage to pursue them."
Walt Disney

READ THIS AGAIN

"Whether you think you can or think you can't, you are usually right."

It's your own personal belief system that is generating results, whether you realize it or not.

You are what you think. Your body does not want or need you to be overweight, so it's not your body that is doing it. It starts in your head.

Your thoughts determine your outcomes because they cause your behaviors.

Once a person is willing to let go of the excuses and the old mindset, possibility opens up.

As a person is willing to recognize the need for change and act in a proactive manner, they unlock the limits.

You have to push a mental re-set button on some things in order to create the possibility of a different outcome.

CHAPTER 7

WHAT COMES FIRST?

Occasionally I meet someone who comes to me for weight loss and it becomes clear that their self-esteem or self-worth is so tragically low that it needs to be addressed before even beginning to deal with the issues of food or exercise. This is because if a person does not really value themselves then they will find themselves unworthy of self care, which includes eating right and exercising appropriately, certainly for any sustainable amount of time. This is one reason why weight loss can be so complicated.

Caring for your body is an act of self love. Neglecting your body is not. It's not simply a matter of a food craving or the lack of motivation to exercise, but rather it's the underlying factors that can determine those behaviors which affect how we treat ourselves. If someone doesn't value themselves they will not value self care.

The lack of self care can manifest itself into a variety of health and weight issues. While a person with low self esteem can often temporarily participate in exercise or go on a diet, they will almost always ultimately fail because the change is being prompted by an external factor rather than an internal factor, thus the changes are perceived as effort and the work required is soon pushed aside with any reasonable although often illogical excuse. Bottom line, a person needs to value themselves enough to regard the acts of eating right and exercising appropriately as positive and deserved self care. Self care is an act of love. One needs to feel deserving of that love, and realize that there's a huge difference between healthy levels of self love versus narcissism and selfishness.

So where does one begin? Perhaps a person should take the time to ask themselves where they are on the priority list of life. Maybe a person should ask themselves if they think they are worth the time it takes to create change. Maybe a person should stop and ask themselves if they love themselves enough to deserve to be thin and healthy. Ignoring these issues can ultimately lead to failure if not addressed and corrected.

There's no point lying about it or sugar coating the facts. Changing eating habits is a process. Learning how to exercise at the appropriate frequency, duration, and intensity and sticking to it consistently takes effort and takes time. Making peace with that fact can only come into play when one realizes that the nurturing of oneself is a selfless rather than selfish act. This has to be important to you. You have to realize that YOU are important enough to do this for yourself.

Making Yourself a Priority

Prioritizing oneself seems to be extremely difficult for some people. Women, parents and caregivers seem to flow into this category quite frequently although not exclusively. Basically, some people seem to put everyone else's needs ahead of their own. Everyone and everything else gets their time and there seems to be no time left over for personal indulgences. Even though self care is hardly an "indulgence", it can be perceived as such by someone who gives all of their time away to others.

It's extremely common for people to tell me that they don't have time to exercise or that they don't have time to shop and prepare their meals because they are too busy with work or tending to the needs of other people in their lives. The truth is they are either not as organized as they believe themselves to be, they don't value themselves enough, they don't really want to put in the work, or they think that it is selfish to take time for themselves in this way. So let's look at these pitfalls:

Time Organization

Often times when people perceive themselves as being so busy that they can't spend the time they need for proper self care, it's often actually a lack of organization and time management or procrastination which can make someone feel as though they're always running behind or too busy. One of the questions I like to ask someone who uses time as an excuse is whether or not they watch TV or spend recreational time on the computer. If the answer is yes, they obviously have time but are choosing to prioritize other things over their health. If the answer is no, then they're likely to benefit by learning some time management or organizational skills. Even then, if someone is truly well organized and simultaneously have truly managed to have scheduled themselves so tightly that they absolutely have zero free time, then it is often a matter of placing themselves at the bottom of the priority list.

People Who Don't Value Themselves Enough

This goes back to the self-esteem and self-worth issue. If a person doesn't value themselves, then they simply won't prioritize themselves. When a person values themselves, they understand the need to respect and respond to their own personal needs and place themselves on their daily priority list.

People who Don't Really Want to Put in the Work

These are the people who create the illusion of being very busy or who actually make themselves very busy in order to have an excuse or even to gain sympathy for their (perceived) inability to take the time to exercise or to eat properly. This may sound harsh on my part, but that it is still a fact, like it or not.

There are a lot of reasons why people avoid exercise and eating right that have nothing to do with time restraints. The real reasons may indeed be absolutely legitimate, but the "time" excuse is readily accepted by both the individual and the people in their life. Thus, a "lack of time" is one of the most common excuses for a lack of self care, whether or not that is the actual truth of the matter.

People who Think it's Selfish to Spend Time on Themselves

This is usually the case when someone is in a demanding personal relationship or has children or other family members to care for. They tend to put other people's needs in front of their own on a regular basis. They also tend to lack the ability to say "no" without feeling guilty. They can find themselves overwhelmed with work projects, social engagements,

PTA involvements, school activities, taxiing others to and fro, amongst other things.

For example, they seem to be under the belief that if they don't witness every one of their kid's soccer games or if they fail to run their children around to a multitude of extracurricular activities they're somehow a bad parent. These people are usually exhausted because they "give and give and give" to others and neglect to give to themselves. Ironically, if they would take the time for themselves to exercise and eat right then they would actually have *more* energy when it comes time to care for others.

A person who is "exhausted" is usually far less engaging than a person with energy. Self care is not selfish at all, and it benefits everyone around that person. Once a person prioritizes themselves and begins to see self care as actually selfless, then they are actually much more productive with others.

Time Whine

If I appear to be unsympathetic to the "time" excuse, it's because I am. The point is that a lot of this is about attitude and being honest...*really honest* with yourself about what is really holding you back. It's about taking a good long look at the nature of the real problem and then making a decision to move past it. There's no point in feeling bad or guilty about any excuses or decisions you may have made in the past with regards to your self-care. Everyone has their reasons at the time. The important part is that we recognize it for what it is, we take action, and we move on.

COMMON REASONS PEOPLE FAIL AT WEIGHT LOSS

A Big Losing Lack of Patience

Many people who are trying to lose weight want to solve their weight problem rapidly. Nobody went to bed thin and healthy and then weirdly woke up with a genuine weight problem. In reality it took weeks, months, and even years to gain the weight and it will take weeks, months, or even years to lose the weight too! In fact, rapid weight loss is practically a sure formula for relapse and weight gain. It's a matter of physiology, but we'll get into that later.

People have been duped into believing that rapid weight loss is a good thing, when the truth is that it can be very harmful from both a physical standpoint and an emotional standpoint. It's time to get real, and real weight loss requires looking at the big picture.

It's no wonder why people get confused. For many years there was a television show with weight loss contestants and they would lose 5-10 pounds a week in the pursuit of a large cash prize. Unfortunately, the show made rapid weight loss appear to be a positive thing. The show didn't truly show the whole picture or show how contestants on that show exercises for several hours a day under the direction of a trainer, had a staff of doctors, nutritionists, and cooks. It also didn't show how much time the contestants spent in the medical and training recovery room each day, being taped up, iced down, and evaluated for injuries. The people on that show were on a very specific and controlled diet and are away from their real life. They were away from work, family, kids, normal life stresses and so on. They literally have nothing else to distract them, not to mention the winner is rewarded with a very large cash prize at the end of the show and will probably make some television appearances and maybe even get an endorsement deal for some diet product. It's mostly surreal. The conditions of this television show were completely unrealistic when compared to the average person's (who is not on television show) life, situations, and predicaments. In fact, a good number of people who lost weight on that show gained part or all of the weight back after the show ended, including the "winner" of the show.

There were a few follow-up stories on these contestants after the fact. The Today Show aired a story called *"Life After "Loser: Every Day is a Struggle,"* where *"the participants of the show reveal that keeping the weight off is a big battle."* In fact, the season 1 winner gained back all the weight he lost on the show. For the first few months, staying active was easy, but when the realities of managing work and family crept it, he found it too demanding. *"I lost the focus I had gained on the show,"* he said. *"And when I started gaining the weight back, I felt guilty."* He said that he went on the show for the right reasons, but a lot of his motivation came from the competition and prospect of winning $250,000.

Additionally, the show never once mentioned how or why the human body was losing weight this fast, and why once the season was over, the weight would come back.

Losing Weight For Real

I've seen it time and time again where people are disappointed that they've *only* lost one or 2 pounds during a week when in fact 1 or 2 pounds is absolutely healthy and desired! Media has managed to convince people that losing large amounts of weight is the indicator of success, whether or not that is actually healthy, or more importantly, whether or not it will have a long-term successful outcome. Hence, the lack of patience is fostered from a number of forces. Not only do we tend to be a very impatient society overall and have become very accustomed to instant gratification, there is also a very general lack of understanding about how the body actually functions and what it really takes to make changes in one's attitude towards food choices and activity levels for the long haul. It takes understanding and patience to lose weight. No one gained a weight problem overnight, so no one can solve a weight problem overnight either!

Rate of Fat Metabolism

The body can only metabolize 2-3 pounds a week of fat. Yes. Read that again.

A measurement of energy expended by the body over a period of time represents the metabolic rate. The basal metabolic rate (BMR) is the rate at which energy is expanded by the body per unit time under controlled conditions. Your BMR (metabolism), is the energy (measured in calories) expended by the body at rest to maintain normal bodily functions. The basal metabolic rate represents the minimal energy required for the work of respiration, digestion, circulation, body temperature regulation, and other activities of the body when the individual is awake. The basal metabolic rate is influenced by a number of factors including hormones, body size, weight, age, gender, diet, exercise habits, environmental temperature, and body temperature.

Because of the increased activity of cellular division, the younger the person is, the higher (faster) the metabolism. A person who is taller and heavier will also tend to have a faster metabolism. However, weight loss becomes more difficult for them as their BMR decreases. Men usually have a greater percentage of lean muscle tissue, so men generally have a 10-15% faster BMR than women. Therefore, it is generally easier and faster for men to lose weight. As a general rule, aim to lose about 8 ounces - 2 pounds a week if you're a woman, and 1-3 pounds if you're a man. This is only a general guideline. You might lose less at times. Pay attention to other changes, such as clothes fitting looser, more energy, better attitude, better sleep, and so on.

All Weight Loss is Not Equal

When we lose weight we don't just lose fat. We lose a combination of body fat, muscle tissue, and cellular hydration. For example, studies show that when we diet, the weight we lose is an average 75% fat and 25% muscle. Additionally, a high percentage of this weight loss is likely to be water loss. Remember, water accounts for about 70% of the total body weight of an average person, with muscle tissue containing approximately 75% water (plus 20% protein and 5% minerals). Body fat contains about 50% water. What this tells us is that if the human body can only metabolize 2-3 pounds of fat in a week then a person should be *concerned* rather than elated when they lose more than 2-3 pounds in that time frame. Even if physiology wasn't your forte, logic would tell you that the additional fat loss had to come from muscle and water loss.

So why care? Because the last thing anyone who is trying to lose weight needs is to lose muscle mass! Resting metabolic rate is increased when one gains muscle mass. While the energy expenditure per pound of lean body mass does not change, the addition of more muscle mass means higher energy expenditure or increased metabolism at rest. By increasing lean muscle mass, the metabolism will increase and aid in the weight-loss process. This means that the more muscle mass you have, the higher your metabolism is and the more fuel (calories) you burn. Muscle loss slows down your BMR and makes it *harder* to lose weight. Even if you do lose weight, if not done with muscle mass conservation and muscle increase in mind, you are highly susceptible to gaining all of the weight back, and usually more. Your goal should be to lose body fat and body fat ONLY.

It's sad when a person is disappointed when they have "only" lost 15 pounds over the course of 3 months or so, even though that is actually perfect! Rather than celebrating, they feel let down. The only thing that let them down was the diet industry, for failing to be honest about what legitimate weight loss looks like.

Chronic dieters have usually been through the process of rapid weight loss before and want the same quick results, only this time permanently. What they failed to realize was that their failure wasn't because of a lack of will power but rather the lack of understanding for the body's physiology.

There will always be plenty of dieters seeking easy solutions and quick fixes. It saddens me when people lose weight too fast, or when people lose a healthy and appropriate amount and become upset, frustrated and discouraged that the scale "only" went down a pound or two. This is a common and destructive attitude that comes from years of chronic diet advertising. Our subconscious minds have been bomb-barded with fallacies about weight loss to the point where many people will feel like failures even when they are on the right track. The conscious as well as the subconscious mind often needs re-educating.

The truth is that patience and a good dose of scientific reality in the form of education about basic anatomy and physiology goes a long way in terms of producing a successful, long-term outcome. This is a case where "the truth will set you free."

READ THIS AGAIN

Caring for your body is an act of self-love.

The more muscle mass you have, the higher your metabolism and the more calories you burn.

The truth is that patience and a good dose of scientific reality in the form of education about basic anatomy and physiology goes a long way in terms of producing a successful, long-term outcome.

As a general rule, aim to lose about 8 ounces - 2 pounds a week if you're a woman, and 1-3 pounds if you're a man.

It takes understanding and patience to lose weight.

CHAPTER 8

NO MORE DIETING

Make Healthy, Balanced Food Choices

We need to consume the right amount of calories. In order to lose weight, your body needs to be working efficiently. This is not possible if your diet does not provide sufficient nutrition. Unhealthy diet habits make your body and your metabolism sluggish and make it harder to lose weight. Beware of fasts, liquid diets, and diets that eliminate entire food groups. Healthy weight loss includes foods from all food groups in reasonable amounts. Eat too little and your body will ultimately want to reserve your calories, making it more difficult to lose weight. Eat too much and the scale will keep climbing!

Our bodies were designed with a survival mechanism in place just in case there is a time of famine. Because of this mechanism, it is easier for the body to store fat. If a person goes on a calorie deficit diet, the body's metabolism decreases in order to conserve energy. In this mode, it is much easier for the body to store what we eat as body fat and burn energy from muscle tissue. Since muscle tissue burns a higher amount of calories, the less we have of it the lower our metabolism will be.

If you lose enough muscle through chronic dieting, lack of resistance training, and/or age related muscle loss, your metabolism will become sluggish and you may end up having to consume very few calories just to maintain your weight. This explains why some overweight people can maintain high body weights even though they consume very little calories.

How Many Calories?

A calorie is simply a unit of measurement in terms of energy. A calorie is not a "bad" thing. It's only a measurement tool, just like a ruler. You use a ruler to measure distance and a calorie to measure energy. It takes 3500 calories to equal 1 pound.

Technically, there is no magic number of calories we should eat each day to lose weight, because it's relative to many variables. It is well known that cutting calories too much slows down the metabolic rate, decreases thyroid output and causes loss of lean mass, so the question is how much of a deficit do you need? There is a threshold where further reductions in calories will have detrimental effects.

If you decide to count calories, the general rule is to not go lower than 1200 calories a day if you are a female, or lower than 1500 calories per day if you are a male. Less than that, and your metabolism is bound to SLOW down. There are a few exceptions to these numbers. For example, if a woman is less than 5 feet tall and just has a little weight to lose, it might be appropriate for her to have less than 1200 calories, but it will still depend on several variables.

You can get more specific if you calculate what your current basal metabolic rate (BMR) is and then by subtracting a certain amount of calories in order to create a deficit which leads to weight loss.

Estimating Your Caloric Needs & BMR

To estimate how many calories you should consume in order to *maintain your weight*, there is a formula called the Harris-Benedict principle that can help you can determine your basal metabolic rate (BMR). Keep in mind, all formulas, including this one, are *estimates*. Remember that there are other factors that influence your BMR such as diet, hormones, and temperature which are not taken into account in these types of calculations. Consider them to be good starting points, but have flexibility in mind. You may need to adjust your numbers according to how your body responds. Everyone's different, and all tools are only relative to their usefulness to the individual. The formula to calculate approximate BMR is as follows (please note that this formula applies only to adults):

Women:
655 + (4.3 x weight in pounds) + (4.7 x height in inches) - (4.7 x age in years)

Men:

66 + (6.3 x weight in pounds) + (12.9 x height in inches) - (6.8 x age in years)

Next, in order to calculate activity into your daily caloric needs, do the following calculation:

- If you are sedentary : BMR x 20 percent
- If you are lightly active: BMR x 30 percent
- If you are moderately active (You exercise most days a week.): BMR x 40 percent
- If you are very active (You exercise intensely on a daily basis or for prolonged periods.): BMR x 50 percent
- If you are extra active (You do hard labor or are in athletic training.): BMR x 60 percent

Add *this number* to your BMR. This will be the number of calories you can eat every day and *maintain* your current weight.

In order to *lose* weight, you'll need to take in fewer calories than this result. As you lose weight, you will need to re-calculate the formula to assess your new BMR.

The equation to reduce body fat is simple: one must burn more calories than one consumes. The laws of physics, which is undeniable, requires the human body (with a normal metabolism) to burn 3500 calories in order to lose one pound of body fat.

In order to lose 1 pound per week, you have to consume 500 less calories per day than you burn. To lose two pounds per week you have to consume 1000 less calories daily than you burn. You have to create a deficit through diet and/or exercise. Beyond this amount of weight loss you run the risk of losing muscle mass, especially if you are female, which makes you feel tired and diminishes your metabolism. This means in order to burn 5, 7, 10, 12 or more pounds of body fat per week (and just body fat) based on your BMR and deficits without having a negative effect is pretty much impossible.

Calorie Counting

Of course, all of this requires calorie counting which may or may not be suitable for everyone. For some people it makes losing weight too much of a hassle and causes them to throw in the towel. Other people find calorie counting a useful tool to help keep them on track and to better understand the foods that they consume. Left brain, number oriented people may tend to find calorie counting useful because the structure is appealing to them.

I typically recommend calorie counting at least during the initial phases if for no other reason than to create more of an *awareness* of what is being consumed. Many people are surprised when they discover that their morning muffin had the caloric equivalent of a large order of fries. Introducing calorie counting can be one way for a person to become more educated about the foods that they eat. However in most cases, I recommend calorie counting or food journaling for limited periods of time. Remember, the goal is to eat healthy naturally, automatically, as part of a long-term lifestyle change. This means that we shouldn't be tracking calories for the long-term either. Once a person has a basic understanding of food and a basic understanding of their body's personal caloric needs, calorie counting or food journaling becomes absolutely unnecessary, as it should be. That's one of the indicators of having a healthy relationship and understanding of food.

Stop Dieting. Choose a Healthy Way of Eating for Life.

Strict diet programs are nearly impossible to follow for the long term. It's easier to learn how to choose healthy foods and decide to choose those foods 90% or more of the time. Don't spend your life dieting. Do it once and do it properly. *This is a new way of eating for life!*

Sensible eating habits have absolutely nothing to do with dieting or having a diet mentality. Most of it boils down to common sense, meaning if you eat too much fat you will be too fat, and if you eat the right amount of lean foods you are likely to be the right amount of lean. This doesn't mean that a healthy, lean person never consumes sugary or fatty foods. The truth of the matter is there will be plenty of Christmas cookies, birthday cakes, and fast food runs during the course of most people's lives and all of these things can be part of the healthy diet as long as they're in the correct ratio when looking at the overall big picture of a person's eating habits. If a person chooses their foods from a place of wisdom the majority of time, the occasional less healthy food choice becomes insignificant in terms of overall weight loss or weight maintenance.

Diets based on deprivation can end up fostering guilt, frustration, or internal rebellion. The emotion or feeling of guilt can cause people to feel like a failure. That feeling of failure tends to be very de-motivating, and the negative emotional toll can override any positive accomplishments. So, you want to have an occasional cookie or an order of French fries? Have it! It's more of a matter of what we choose on a regular basis.

Be Prepared for Less Than Perfect Days

Every day might not be a day filled with smart foods and exercise. If you have a less than perfect day, don't give up! If you get off track, just recognize it and get right back on track. Don't delay. All is not lost! Just start right back up again. A quick recovery is the best way to keep a positive attitude.

Eat Often Enough

Many people fall into the trap of allowing themselves to go hungry. What happens? They get tired, crabby, and unhappy. What happens then? They reach for whatever is quickly available or even binge eat. See what I mean? Hunger is a disaster! Avoid it.

Good food decisions and eating patterns will increase and speed up your metabolism. It is important to avoid skipping meals and in some cases to eat healthy snacks in-between meals (Yes, snacking is okay if you are actually hungry). The idea is to eat frequently enough to prevent strong hunger pangs and to keep your energy levels consistent.

Many dieters have been taught to believe that snacking is a negative thing. While it's true that improper snacking is a negative thing, there is such a thing as *proper snacking*. For example, eating high fat and high sugar foods out of a vending machine is not the same as choosing an apple as an in-between meal snack. The choice of snack will have entirely different outcomes especially when repeated in any sort of habitual sense.

While comparing a candy bar to an apple seems like common sense in terms of snacking choices, in some cases the "dieter's" subconscious mind views all snacks in the same light. Here is another case where education becomes detrimental not only for the conscious mind, but for the subconscious mind as well. As the conscious and subconscious mind can come to an understanding that certain snack choices are actually beneficial for weight loss, then any negative ideas or beliefs harbored in the subconscious mind can be released. So being specific matters. Once a person understands what "healthy" snacks means and they understand *when* healthy snacks are appropriate, then it becomes important to reinforce to the subconscious mind that appropriate healthy snacking is a positive behavior. This has to coincide with appropriate nutritional education, as well as tuning into the fact of whether or not the body actually needed a snack. One way to do this is to tune into your body's signals.

Assess the Body's Signals

People often confuse dropping energy levels with hunger and will eat when sometimes food is not the actual issue. While indeed changing the blood sugar levels can cause a person to feel tired, sometimes the actual cause for fatigue is stress, dehydration, or a lack of proper sleep. Another common contributor pertains to the individual who consumes a lot of caffeinated products. Sometimes when a person is accustomed to having a stimulated central nervous system via the intake of caffeine, they may begin to perceive that they are fatigued when in actuality their central nervous system is settling down into normal ranges as the caffeine wears off.

I believe that it is important to assess the reasons why one chooses unplanned eating. In some cases there will be a legitimate need for food and a legitimate need for the food to help stabilize blood sugar levels. But in the case of unplanned food, one should ask themselves, "Why am I eating this? Am I hungry? Am I tired? Am I stressed? Am I thirsty?"

Often times the best thing to do is to drink a glass of water first. Sometimes thirst can cause fatigue or disguise itself as hunger, and you might not even be hungry at all. Wait 20 minutes, and if you're still starting to feel hungry, then eat. Even if stress is a cause, often the act of removing oneself from the situation (either emotionally or physically) while getting a glass of water can give a mental reprieve. Obviously, if there is an ongoing stressor it should be dealt with, especially if it causes negative or self-destructive behaviors.

If you are tired, think about why that may be the case. Are you getting enough sleep? Have you been undergoing a lot of physical, emotional, or mental activity lately? Have you become dependent upon caffeine? The answer to these questions determines what the response should be, taking note that food is typically not the answer here.

Are you actually hungry? If so, it's a good idea to eat!

Reconnecting to Your Body

All of this is ultimately going to be about you having good information about your body and what it needs to function properly while establishing a strong connection to your body and the messages it's sending you. Your body is wise. It's been communicating with you the whole time. It's time to hear its wisdom. It's time to reconnect.

READ THIS AGAIN

Eat too little and your body will ultimately want to reserve your calories, making it more difficult to lose weight. Eat too much and the scale will keep climbing!

If you lose enough muscle through chronic dieting, lack of resistance training, and/or age related muscle loss, your metabolism will become sluggish and you may end up having to consume very few calories just to maintain your weight.

It is important to assess the reasons why one chooses unplanned eating. One should ask themselves, "Why am I eating this? Am I hungry? Am I tired? Am I stressed? Am I thirsty?"

Sensible eating habits have absolutely nothing to do with dieting.

If you get off track, just recognize it and get right back on track.

Good food decisions and eating patterns will increase and speed up your metabolism.

there is no magic number of calories we should eat each day to lose weight, because it's relative to many variables.

If you decide to count calories, the general rule is to not go lower than 1200 calories a day if you are a female, or lower than 1500 calories per day if you are a male.

Your body is wise. It's been communicating with you the whole time. It's time to hear its wisdom. It's time to reconnect.

CHAPTER 9

FOOD 101

Food is simply fuel. Some of it is high quality fuel and some of it is low quality fuel. Some of it will make your body feel wonderful and be the amazing gift that we get to live in. Other choices can cause the body to break down and cause the body to feel like a prison.

In order to feel our best and carry the correct amount of weight for our frame, we need to have a basic understanding of what foods are composed of. Once we do, the craziness of diets will seem….well…crazy. Most importantly, you will be fully empowered to redesign your body based on your choices.

To do that, what we simply need to do is to look at foods based on what they do for us and how our bodies react to them. So let's start at the beginning.

Protein

Protein is a key component of every cell in the body. Hair and nails are mostly made of protein. Your body uses protein to build and repair tissues, including muscle recovery and repair. It does *not* build muscle (exercise does that), but it is needed to help the body build muscle in conjunction with exercise. You also need protein to make enzymes, hormones, and other body chemicals.

Protein Examples:
Best: Chicken or turkey breast (no skin), cod (most white fish), dried beans/legumes, egg whites, lean Meats, non-fat cottage cheese, non-fat yogurt, skim milk, organic tofu, veggie burgers/sausage, powdered peanut butter, etc.
Less often: Turkey bacon, 1% milk, chicken or turkey dark meat (no skin), part-skim mozzarella cheese, peanut butter (no sugar, low fat), salmon,

sharp cheddar cheese, tuna (packed in water), whole eggs, nuts (very sparingly as they are very high in fat), etc.

Mostly avoid: Bacon, cream, half & half, high fat cheese (colby, jack, etc.), organ meats, whole milk, etc.

Protein is slower to digest and will help you feel fuller longer. If your appetite and actual hunger cause you to *overeat*, look for ways to increase your protein.

Protein is an important building block of bones, muscles, cartilage, skin, and blood. Protein is a "macronutrient," meaning that the body needs relatively large amounts of it. The body does not store protein, and therefore has no reserve to draw on when it needs a new supply. However, the body will cannibalize its own muscle tissue for protein if it needs to in order to protect itself. The body was designed to sacrifice some tissues in order to protect more vital tissues.

Believe it or not, diets can actually force the body into these modes which is dangerous and unhealthy. The body needs a certain amount of protein but not an excessive amount. High-protein/low-carbohydrate diets have been around for years. When people eat a lot of protein but few carbohydrates, their metabolisms change into a state called ketosis. Ketosis means the body converts from burning carbohydrates for fuel to burning its own fat. When fat is broken down, bits of carbon called ketones are released into the bloodstream as energy sources. Ketosis, which also happens in diabetes, tends to suppress appetite, causing people to eat less, and it also increases the body's elimination of fluids through urine, resulting in a loss of water weight. While this may sound like a good thing, ketosis can become dangerous when ketones build up. High levels lead to dehydration and change the chemical balance of your blood to become too acidic. If blood becomes acidic it can damage the kidneys, liver, and brain. Additionally, the body produces ammonia when it breaks down protein. Nobody knows the long-term risks of higher levels of ammonia in the body.

There is also evidence to suggest that people who eat high-protein diets tend to excrete excess calcium in their urine. This suggests that the body is releasing calcium into the bloodstream to counteract an increase in acids caused by too much protein consumption. Calcium loss could lead to osteoporosis.

Some of the other side-effects of high-protein/low carbohydrate diets are mental fogginess, poor mood control, bad breath, and "keto-crotch" (strong, unpleasant odors emanating from your crotch).

This "high-protein" diet mentality trades short-term benefits for long-term health consequences.

Bottom line: Protein is important! However, high protein/low carbohydrate based diets are potentially dangerous AND completely unnecessary in order to lose weight.

Some people get wrapped up into the smallest details and want to know how many specific grams of protein they need, which of course, varies tremendously. Once you start eating out of all of the food groups and paying attention to your body's feedback, your body will give you the answer. The simplest strategy is to have some lean protein with each meal, and include complex carbohydrates. Yes, I just wrote that down. *Include* carbohydrates. Read on.

Carbohydrates

Carbohydrates have been unfairly villanized by the diet industry. Carbohydrates have been all lumped into the same category, however there are different types of carbohydrates. The different types are very, very different from each other, and it is important to know the differences because some types of carbohydrate are needed for the body to function properly, while other types are totally unnecessary or harmful.

Carbohydrates are macronutrients and are the body's main source of energy. They are called carbohydrates because, at the chemical level, they contain carbon, hydrogen and oxygen. All macronutrients must be obtained through diet; the body cannot produce macronutrients on its own.

Carbohydrates provide fuel for the central nervous system and energy for muscles. They also prevent protein from being used as an energy source and enable fat metabolism. Additionally, carbohydrates are important for brain function, and are the brain's primary source of fuel. Carbohydrates influence mood, memory, decision-making, and focus.

Simple carbohydrates contain just one or two sugars. They can be found in dairy products, candy, soda, syrups, fruit, beer, cakes, etc.

Simple carbohydrates digest quickly and have a fast impact on blood sugar levels. However, the simple carbohydrates from an apple and the simple carbohydrates from a candy bar do not make these choices equal.

Carbohydrates that are made with processed and refined sugars and do not have vitamins, minerals or fiber are called "empty calories" and can lead to weight gain and cause rapid spikes in blood sugar. In contrast, simple carbohydrates that are found in nature (like the apple), contain fiber and are nutrient dense. In other words, the apple has value to the body and the candy bar stresses the body. One can cause problems. One will not.

Some categorize fruit as being a complex carbohydrate, since fruit is actually a mix of carbohydrates. Fruit contains natural fruit sugar (fructose is a simple carbohydrate) as well as dietary fiber (also a type of carbohydrate). The most healthful carbohydrates are unrefined plants that are low in sugars and high in fiber. So is fruit a simple or complex carb? Are potatoes bad for you too? Hold that thought, and let's dig into the carb category a little deeper.

Complex carbohydrates such as rice, peas, pasta, grains, etc. are good for sustaining energy and mental focus. Complex carbohydrates are helpful for your body. Avoiding complex carbohydrates can be trendy, but it is a mistake.

Complex carbohydrates, in contrast to simple carbohydrates can keep you full longer and keep blood sugar levels steady, especially when eaten with protein.

Foods that are mostly made up of simple carbohydrates, such as candy, pastries, and soda, provide a quick source of energy, but they are digested quickly and spike your blood sugar. Complex carbohydrates take longer to break down since their molecular structure is larger. Carbohydrates rich in fiber move slowly through the digestive tract, and help us to feel fuller for longer, so it can help prevent over eating.

Fiber is another form of carbohydrate. There are two types of fiber that your body needs: soluble and insoluble. Both come from plants and are forms of carbohydrates. Unlike other food components, such as fats, proteins, or simple or complex carbohydrates, which your body breaks down and absorbs, fiber can't be broken down and absorbed by your digestive system. Instead, it moves through your body relatively intact which slows digestion and makes your stools softer and easier to pass. This helps with weight loss because high-fiber foods tend to be more filling than low-fiber foods, so you're more likely to eat less and stay full longer. Additionally, high-fiber foods tend to have fewer calories for the same volume of food.

Fiber benefits go way beyond weight control and healthy digestion. It also helps lower cholesterol, stabilizes blood sugar, and even helps keep you alive longer by reducing cholesterol. Increasing your dietary fiber intake may reduce the risk of dying from cardiovascular disease and cancer.

Most fiber filled foods contain both insoluble and soluble fiber but usually contain more of one type than the other.

Soluble fiber dissolves in water to form a gel-like material. It can help reduce blood cholesterol and glucose levels. Soluble fiber is found in foods such as oats, peas, beans, apples, blueberries, citrus fruits, carrots, barley and psyllium.

Insoluble fiber promotes the movement of material through your digestive system and increases stool bulk, so it can be useful to those who have constipation, hemorrhoids, bowel incontinence, or irregular stools. It is found in whole wheat flour, wheat bran, nuts, brown rice, fruit and vegetable skins, beans and vegetables, such as cauliflower, green beans and potatoes, amongst other foods.

Love, Logic & Carbs.

So, are carbohydrates such as potatoes and fruit good for you or bad for you? In all of my years in this industry, I have *never* met anyone that had a weight issue due to too much produce in their diet… ever. Eat them. Please.

Do low and no carb diets make sense? Absolutely not. This does not mean we should eat carbohydrates without any restraint. Remember, simple and complex carbohydrates provide *energy*, but if you eat more "energy" than you spend, your body will store the excess as fat. Therefore, carbohydrate consumption should be based on *energy usage*. This basically means that if you are active, your body needs more carbohydrates than if you are sedentary.

Carbohydrate Examples:
Best: Brown rice, fruits and vegetables, oatmeal (not pre-packaged), vegetable juice, whole wheat pasta, whole or sprouted grain breads, etc.
Less often: Fruit juice, white pasta, white rice, white breads, etc.
Mostly avoid: Chips, crackers, ramen type noodles, soda, alcohol, candy, pastry, ice cream, and other sugar based items, etc.

Fat

Fats have a purpose, however they are calorie dense (so it's easy to overdo) and your body can only use fat as FAT. Try to use healthier fats vs. less healthy varieties when you *have* to use or consume fat. Otherwise, avoid it. Think about it this way, when you endeavor to lose weight, you are actually

71

trying to lose *fat*... so stop adding to it. Even "healthy" foods can be turned into "unhealthy" foods if cooked in too much fat.

You don't have to eliminate all fat from your diet. In fact, some vitamins are fat soluble so fats can actually help promote good health. But there are different types of fat to be aware of, and we want to take note on the amount of fat we consume.

Fat Facts

There are different types of fat. Your body makes its own fat if you consume excess calories. Dietary fats are found in foods.

As babies and toddlers, fat is needed for brain development, but I'm assuming you are over the age of two if you are reading this, so this is no longer an issue.

Fat plays a role in skin, hair, hormones, organ protection, satiation, and nutrient utilization. This is taken care of by consuming the correct amount of dietary fat and having enough essential fat on our bodies. For women, this is around 13% body fat and around 5% for men, although some people needs are higher than that.

Some types of dietary fat can play a role in cardiovascular disease. Fats are high in calories (9 calories per gram) when compared gram to gram with proteins and carbohydrates (4 calories per gram), so you need to monitor your fat intake against the other foods you eat so that you don't take in more calories than you need. If you eat more calories than you need, you will gain weight.

Unhealthy fats

There are two main types of harmful dietary fats:

- **Saturated fat.** This type of fat comes mostly from animal sources. Saturated fats raise high-density lipoprotein (HDL or "good") cholesterol and low-density lipoprotein (LDL or "bad") cholesterol levels, which can increase your risk of cardiovascular disease.

- **Trans fat.** Most trans fats are made from oils through a food processing method called partial hydrogenation. Partially hydrogenated trans fats can increase total blood cholesterol, LDL ("bad") cholesterol and triglyceride levels, but lower HDL ("good") cholesterol. This can raise your risk of cardiovascular disease.

Most saturated fats or trans fats are solid at room temperature. They include animal fat, coconut oil, shortening, butter, and stick margarine.

Healthier fats

The potentially helpful types of dietary fat are primarily unsaturated fats:

- **Monounsaturated fatty acids and Polyunsaturated fatty acids.** Foods with monounsaturated fatty acids and/or polyunsaturated fatty acids instead of saturated fats can help improve blood cholesterol levels, decrease your risk of heart disease, and may also help reduce the risk of type 2 diabetes.
- **Omega-3 fatty acids.** Omega-3, found in some types of fatty fish, appears to decrease the risk of coronary artery disease. Fish high in omega-3 fatty acids include salmon, tuna, trout, mackerel, sardines and herring. There are also krill and plant sources of omega-3 fatty acids. Plant sources of omega-3 fatty acids include flaxseed (ground), oils (canola, flaxseed, soybean), winter squash, and nuts and other seeds (walnuts, pecans, hemp seeds, pumpkin seeds, and chia seeds).

Fats made up mostly of monounsaturated and polyunsaturated fats are liquid at room temperature, such as canola oil, olive oil, avocado oil, safflower oil, peanut oil, sunflower oil and corn oil.

Recommendations for fat intake

Because some fats are potentially helpful and others are potentially harmful to your health, and *both* can lead to weight gain, it's important to know which ones you are eating and how much. Here's the main points:

- Avoid trans fat. Check food labels and look for the amount of trans fat listed and/or the words "partially hydrogenated."

73

- Replace harmful fats with healthier fats.
- Use oil instead of solid fats. For example, use olive oil instead of butter.
- Include omega-3 rich fish in your food choices. Bake, poach, or broil seafood instead of frying it.
- Choose lean meat and skinless poultry.
- Limit saturated fat to less than 10 percent of calories a day. For example: a 1500 calorie diet should have less than 150 calories (14 grams) of saturated fat. However, keep in mind that we should be choosing unsaturated fat, and minimizing or avoiding saturated fats.
- For weight loss, *total* fat gram intake should be no more than 45 grams per day. 15-30 grams is better. Less than 15 grams is probably too low. Like all things, the exact amount needed varies from person to person, but this gives you a general idea.

Fat Examples:

Best: Avocado, flax seed oil, most nuts, olive oil, olives, omega-3 sources, etc.

Mostly avoid: Butter, cream cheese, sour cream, fried foods, lard, solid fats, animal-based fats, mayonnaise, etc.

READ THIS AGAIN

Food is simply fuel. Some of it is high quality fuel and some of it is low quality fuel.

You are fully empowered to redesign your body based on your choices.

We simply need to look at foods based on what they do for us and how our bodies react to them.

When people eat a lot of protein but few carbohydrates, their metabolisms change into a state called ketosis. Ketosis can become dangerous when ketones build up.

The simplest strategy is to have some lean protein with each meal, and include complex carbohydrates. Carbohydrates provide fuel for the central nervous system and energy for muscles.

Carbohydrates are important for brain function, and are the brain's primary source of fuel, influencing mood, memory, decision-making, and focus.

The most healthful carbohydrates are unrefined plants that are low in sugars and high in fiber.

Fiber is a form of carbohydrate. Fiber benefits include, weight control, healthy digestion, lower cholesterol, blood sugar stabilization, reducing cholesterol, and reducing the risk of dying from cardiovascular disease and cancer.

Carbohydrate consumption should be based on energy usage.

Most unhealthy fats (saturated and trans fats) are solid at room temperature. Healthier fats (monounsaturated and polyunsaturated fats) are usually liquid at room temperature.

CHAPTER 10

Sugar, Sugar

Why a whole chapter on sugar? Because sugar has an addictive quality to it and can be a real struggle for many people. Most everybody knows that sugar isn't healthy, but just what *is* sugar doing inside of our bodies? What's taking place once we eat it? Most of us think about how the extra calories can pile up on the waistline, but there's more to it...a lot more. Read on and you'll see the sweet stuff really isn't that sweet.

Your Body on Sugar
- When you eat sugar, your blood sugar quickly rises and your pancreas immediately jumps into overdrive. This increase in blood sugar causes the pancreas to secrete the hormone insulin, which is an important hormone in the body. It allows glucose (blood sugar) to enter cells from the bloodstream and tells the cells to start burning glucose instead of fat. If there's no demand for that energy, it gets stored as fat. If it stays in your bloodstream, it becomes a toxic sludge and one of the reasons for diabetes complications, such as blindness. The body tries to counteract this by releasing both adrenaline and cortisol (stress hormones). This chain reaction is a recipe for fat gain disaster and dramatically increases the risk of becoming overweight. Meanwhile, your heart rate may go up higher and you might feel a little flushed or slightly nauseous at this point. Any "sugar highs" are followed by a "sugar crash" when all the sugar is finally out of your bloodstream, causing you to feel sluggish and tired.

Your Immune System on Sugar
- The surge of glucose, insulin, cortisol, and adrenaline can send your immune system into a tailspin. Free radicals have a heyday which lowers your immune system. Excess sugar can cause a drop in the ability of white blood cells to destroy bacteria. Result? You just became more vulnerable to things like the common cold.

- Sugar may increase your risk of certain cancers. Cancer is characterized by uncontrolled multiplication and growth of cells. Insulin is one of the key hormones in regulating this sort of growth. Though studies are not wholly conclusive, some research suggests that excessive added sugar is associated with higher levels of certain cancers, such as pancreatic cancer. Additionally, the metabolic problems linked to sugar consumption are a known contributor of inflammation, another potential cause of cancer.

Your Liver on Sugar

- Sugar can cause fatty liver disease. Sugar cannot be metabolized by the liver in large amounts. This isn't a problem as long as we eat small amounts (like a piece of fruit). Fructose is converted into glycogen and stored in the liver until we need it. However, if the liver is already full of glycogen, the extra sugar can overload the liver, forcing it to convert it into fat and causing the liver to store the fat in unusual places, which can lead to globules of fat building up around your liver. This effect can lead to fatty liver disease, which is a major risk factor for diabetes, heart attacks, and cancer.

- Sugar can lead to insulin resistance, diabetes, and metabolic disorders. When cells become resistant to the effects of insulin, the cells in the pancreas make more of it. Eventually, as insulin resistance gradually becomes worse, the pancreas can't keep up with the demand of making enough insulin to keep blood sugar levels down.

Your Mouth on Sugar

- You've heard this before and it's true. Eating too much sugar can promote cavities and gum disease. Sugar also provides a quick food source for bacteria so they can reproduce quickly, causing plaque buildup and that unpleasant morning breath.

Your Skin on Sugar

- Sugar can age you! Sugar in your bloodstream attaches to proteins to form harmful new molecules called Advanced Glycation End

77

products, or AGEs. These invaders attack nearby proteins, damaging them, including protein fibers in collagen and elastin (the components that keep your skin firm and elastic). The outcome? Sugar can cause dry, brittle protein fibers that lead to wrinkles and saggy, dull skin. AGEs also promote the growth of fragile collagen and deactivate your body's natural antioxidant enzymes, which makes your skin more susceptible to sun damage.

- Sugar also has an effect on the severity of acne because of the hormonal fluctuations it triggers. The inflammation caused by excess sugar has also been linked to other skin conditions, like psoriasis.

Your Heart on Sugar

- There is a strong statistical connection between sugar intake and the risk of heart disease. People with higher sugar intakes have a marked increase in risk of heart attacks compared to those with lower intakes. People who consume a lot of added sugar are more likely to have lower levels of HDL (good cholesterol), higher levels of LDL (bad cholesterol), and higher levels of triglycerides (blood fats). Bad cholesterol and blood fats clog up arteries and blood vessels, leading to heart disease.

- The American Heart Association recommends women only consume 6 teaspoons or 100 calories a day from added sugars, and 9 teaspoons or 150 calories for men. The CDC reports that the average American eats between 13 and 20 teaspoons of added sugar a day. For perspective, an average can of soda contains 12 teaspoons of sugar. There are 4 grams of sugar in 1 teaspoon.

- Sugar can also raise blood pressure. Chronic high insulin levels can cause the smooth muscle cells around each blood vessel to grow faster than normal. This causes tense artery walls, something that puts you on the path to high blood pressure, which increases the workload of the heart and arteries and can cause damage to the whole circulatory system. Eventually, this can lead to heart disease, heart attacks, stroke, kidney damage, artery disease, and other serious coronary conditions.

- People who have diets where at least 25 percent of the calories came from added sugar are twice as likely to die from cardiovascular disease than those who have diets where added sugars make up less than 10 percent of the food they eat .

- Fructose elevates uric acid, which decreases nitric oxide, raises angiotensin, and causes your smooth muscle cells to contract, thereby raising your blood pressure and potentially damaging your kidneys. Increased uric acid also leads to chronic, low-level inflammation.

Your Brain on Sugar

- Type 3 diabetes is a title that has been proposed for Alzheimer's disease which results from resistance to insulin in the brain. There is a link between insulin resistance, high-fat diets, and Alzheimer's disease. In this case, the brain's ability to use glucose and produce energy is damaged.

- A diet high in added sugar reduces the production of a chemical known as brain-derived neurotrophic factor (BDNF), which helps the brain form new memories and remember the past. Levels of BDNF are low in people with an impaired glucose metabolism (diabetics and pre-diabetics) and low BDNF has been linked to dementia and Alzheimer's disease. Research shows that eating too much sugar can cause impair cognitive function and reduce proteins that are needed for memory and responsiveness.

- It's addictive. Sugar triggers the release of chemicals that set off the brain's pleasure center, in this case opioids and dopamine. Just like drugs, people develop a tolerance for sugar. You become "sensitized" to sugar and more sensitive to its toxic effects as well. In rat studies looking at sugar addiction, they experience chattering teeth, tremors, shakes, and anxiety when it's taken away, classic signs of withdrawal.

- Sugar can make you think you are hungry when you are not. Eating too much sugar can scramble your body's ability to tell your brain you're full, because it can cause leptin resistance. Leptin's job is to say, "I'm full!" Over-consumption of sugar also triggers the over production of ghrelin, that signals to your body that it's hungry. As a result, you keep eating without necessarily realizing you're full. Your brain still thinks you're still hungry.

- Sugar is linked to depression. Studies are finding a link between depression and eating sugary and junk foods. After six years, those who ate the most junk faced a 40% greater risk of developing depression. In another study, older adults who drank more than four servings of pop per day were 30% more likely to be diagnosed with depression than people who drank unsweetened drinks.

All Sugars Are Not Equal

Dextrose, fructose, and glucose are all sugars. The primary difference between them is how your body metabolizes them. Glucose is the form of energy you were designed to run on. Every cell in your body uses glucose for energy. If we don't get it from the diet, our bodies produce it. This means that complex carbohydrates are useful when eaten in the correct amounts.

Fructose is different. Our bodies do not produce it in any significant amount and there is no physiological need for it. Keep in mind that this doesn't apply to natural, whole foods, like fruit. It is almost impossible to overeat fructose by eating fruit. Whole fruits contain vitamins, antioxidants, and fiber that *reduce* the hazardous effects of fructose. Fiber is necessary in curbing sugar intake. Basically, fiber and fructose need to work together. Fiber is fructose's useful partner. Fructose helps with sweetness, while fiber helps make fructose useful. So how do you eat fiber with your fructose? Get your fructose from fruit or other sources that contain built-in fiber.

The real problems start up when sugar is added to foods during processing, which is more common than you may realize. Think of processed foods as being items that have been already put together to produce a completed, edible food product, and yes, processed foods are used in restaurants too. There is a crazy amount of added sugar to things, even savory (not obviously sweet) foods.

Processed foods are a Pandora's box of potential problems. The solution? Buy *real* food in the grocery store and prepare it at home. Take control.

It should also go without saying, that obvious sugar sources (candy, cake, chocolate, donuts, etc.) should be avoided or greatly minimized. Unless it's growing naturally, it's probably junk, and the last time I checked I have never seen a donut tree.

It all comes back to a simple premise. *Eat healthier and you'll be healthier.*

READ THIS AGAIN

The surge of glucose, insulin, cortisol, and adrenaline can send your immune system into a tailspin.

Sugar can cause fatty liver disease.

Sugar promotes cavities, gum disease, and bad breath.

Sugar ages your skin.

Sugar affects the severity of acne.

Sugar increases the risk of heart disease.

Sugar can raise blood pressure.

Sugar can cause low-level inflammation.

There is a link to sugar and Alzheimer's.

Sugar can cause you to think you are hungry when you are not.

Sugar is linked to depression.

All sugars are not the same.

CHAPTER 11

THE DIET

There is no diet plan to follow. There *is* an *awareness* of choices to adopt into our eating strategies. So, if you really want a diet to follow, make it **"The *Awareness* Diet"**.

On "The Awareness Diet", you will need to be aware of **what foods consist of** (For example: Are they proteins or carbohydrates? If they are carbohydrates, what type are they?). You will need to be aware of **what foods do** (For example: Fiber helps with digestion and feeling full). You will need to be **aware of the approximate calorie range** you need (look in chapter 8 to figure this out). You will need to be **aware of what your carbohydrate needs are** based on your activity level (active people need more, sedentary people need less). You will need to be **aware of whether or not your food choices are valuable to your body** (an orange has nutritional and nutrient value while a candy bar does not). You will need to be **aware of whether a particular food has a positive or negative interaction with your body** (some people need to avoid certain foods due to intolerance, allergies, or medical conditions). You need to be **aware of the signals the body sends you** (hungry, full, weak, etc.).

This sounds like a lot of awareness, and it is. But it's also the easiest strategy and will always be correct. It's based upon the principles of working directly with your body's physiology without trying to trick or stress the body, like so many diet's do. It's not about deprivation. It's about making informed and intelligent choices with a reasonable amount of consistency. In fact, I could put this diet plan on one page. Oh look, I just did.

CHAPTER 12

THE FITNESS FACTOR

If we start consuming fewer calories, our body notices immediately and starts to slow down the metabolism in order to conserve energy. This can cause our weight loss to slow down too. The best answer to this problem is to boost our energy requirement by exercising.

Exercise burns calories, gives us more energy and helps us reduce our body fat percentage. Result? Weight loss is faster and easier.

You don't have to train like an athlete or pump iron for hours each day, unless of course you want a body that looks like an athlete or a body builder. For most people, a regular 30 minute bout of moderate exercise will accomplish a boost in metabolism, but it must be consistent. Some bodies need more exercise, depending on your current level of fitness. If what you are doing isn't working, that's a very strong indicator that your approach is not working well for your specific body and your specific goals.

Our bodies are uniquely coded and have needs based on that individuality. This means that you might have to experiment with discovering what type, what duration, and what intensity of exercise is the right combination for you.

Aerobic activity burns the most fat, while increasing muscle mass revs up the metabolism. A good program includes both.

I've heard time and time again people tell me, "I've tried exercise before but it just doesn't work for me." The reality is that the *reason* that exercise "didn't work" for them is that they exercised *incorrectly* for their body and their goals, and/or they had unrealistic expectations from what they were doing, or they were simply impatient. There is a definite delayed effect from when we start consistently exercising to when we start to see results.

Exercise absolutely works! Exercise in itself is a science and it takes some finesse to figure out just what combination of exercises at what level of intensity and type of frequency rate produces the desired results. This is why exercise can become such a mind game for some people and causes them to be frustrated and give up. Figuring out the right combination that works is a worthwhile venture but sometimes takes some patience and often needs some guidance. But for the people who are willing to take the steps, the benefits that exercise provides is priceless.

I Resolve to Get in Shape!

It's as predictable as the sun rising and setting each day. If you go to nearly any gym in the country sometime between January 1st and the end of March you will find more machines being used and more exercise classes being attended than any other time of the year. After that, you can expect a steady decline with a significant drop off in the summer, followed by a minor increase in gym usage again in the fall, which will then again decline sharply once the holiday season begins in November. Then, just as the sun rises and sets each day, the gym cycle will continue in January will bring forth another upswing of attendance and a plethora of people with New Year's resolutions vowing to get into shape.

It's easy enough to explain why a typical gym has such a dramatically fluctuating membership numbers, especially between January and March. It all starts with New Year's resolutions. It's one of the times during the year when people make a so-called commitment to change and better themselves. Most of these New Year's resolutions will not ultimately lead to the desired outcome. In part, it is because New Year's resolutions are conscious decisions yet most of the habits and behavior changes require change from a subconscious perspective, which is a fact that many people fail to recognize (But you know that because you read chapters 4,5,and 6, right?). This applies to all resolutions that deal with habit change, but since I am elaborating on the exercise component of weight loss, I will focus on the resolution of, "I will get into shape" since it is a common theme to people trying to lose weight, particularly in January.

Sadly, most people who start habit changes because of a New Year's resolution lack the support, guidance, and internal motivation to continue. They get discouraged and quit.

One way to avoid this is to genuinely consider your reasons for wanting to make a change. Write them down, and go beyond the obvious "To be healthy" reason. That's an excellent reason, but give it some depth. What does being 'healthy' do for you? Would you have more energy? Would you breathe better? Would you fit better in your clothes? Would you improve your odds of avoiding a disease? Would you be able to go hiking, traveling, play with kids, bike, or _____(fill in the blank) better?

Long term weight loss isn't a *temporary* goal, but rather it is a long term (permanent) *perspective change* and application of healthy habits and behaviors as a lifestyle choice. For that reason, you want to look at how the benefits of losing weight the right way can change your life!

One more note. If you are serious, you won't wait until Monday (and binge out all weekend) to make a change, and certainly don't wait until January 1st. Once you genuinely make the decision, begin your new journey. Right then.

Exercise is a Head Game

Exercise is just as much mental as it is physical. Without a good understanding about how the body works from an anatomical and physiological perspective it can be very hard to achieve the desired results, and since exercise can cause physical discomfort and be time consuming, many people stop exercising if there are no benefits being gained, or at least the perception of no benefits.

There are many obstacles to exercise success. Some of those obstacles are real while some of those obstacles are perceptions or a lack of flexibility. So a person really needs to take the time to ask themselves a series of questions before embarking on this particular journey.

Am I willing to accept full responsibility? This means letting go of the excuses. This means it's time to stop falsely blaming genetics, age, other people, or circumstances regarding your history with exercise and weight loss.

This may sound hard to hear and it does not mean that person themselves is a failure. It does however mean their previous *approach* and attitude failed so their previous *approaches* and attitudes were failures. Therefore, a person must be willing to change, adapt, and be willing to take full accountability for their own physical predicament. The person who sits down in my office and tells me that "I've done everything right" in terms of exercise and eating are often the ones in biggest denial, and the most stubborn about it. Obviously! If they had done *"everything right"* they wouldn't have the weight issues they have.

Exercise, fitness, and health are things that cannot be provided or given. They are things only you can do for yourself and it's not until you stop blaming external factors will you truly become empowered. By taking full responsibility of your body you immediately begin a brand new connection with it! Your body is impressive, and it can be re-shaped according to your knowledge, your actions, and your love.

Affirmations that help are:
- ♥ "I am willing to take responsibility for my body."
- ♥ "I am responsible for my body."
- ♥ "I am willing to try new things."
- ♥ "My body is unique to me."
- ♥ "My body works with me to find my personal code for success, so I listen to it."

Are you willing to invest the time? There's no getting around this. Exercise takes time. Depending on the goal of the individual this can be a time investment of several hours a week.

There's a lot of confusion on how much time a person should have to exercise and this confusion leads to frustration when people follow the "recommendations" that do not achieve results. That is because it is impossible to dictate healthy exercise recommendations as a blanket statement to the general population and have it be accurate for everyone. Your body is unique and will have its own unique requirements.

A person with the goal of maintenance has different needs than a person with the goal of weight loss. A person with the goal of achieving a certain look has different needs than a person wanting to achieve increased energy levels. A person looking to decrease joint pain has different needs than a person wanting to compete in a body building contest. The examples go on and on and on.

Exercise time requirements depend solely upon the individual and the individuals goals. Exercise time requirements have little or nothing to do with the typical recommendations offered up to the general public. You might as well consider the most common recommendation of 20 minutes a day, three times a week to be a myth.

The body's ability and efficiency in burning fat is directly linked to activity type, intensity, and duration. Duration means time spent in a particular activity and intensity. If any of those factors are off (mode, intensity, or time) then fat loss as well as other exercise benefits will be minimized. The time commitment needs to be viewed with flexibility as the time commitment requirements will change as the body responds and adapts. This means that a time commitment that may have once worked is no longer valid and one must be willing to accept and adapt accordingly in order to achieve the desired results.

Affirmations that help are:
- ♥ "I am willing to spend the time that is needed for my body."
- ♥ "My body is in a constant state of change and transformation."
- ♥ "I respond to my body's needs."
- ♥ "Spending time exercising my body is important and wise."
- ♥ "I deserve to spend time with my body to give it its movement needs."

Are you willing to exercise at the correct intensity? If you're just starting out, take it slow and gradually increase your activity over time. The tendency is to suddenly be motivated and work out too much in the beginning (as with the typical New Year's resolution exerciser). This usually just makes the average person tired and sore, which makes exercise seem less appealing and increases your chances of dropping out. Also, doing too much too soon drains energy, while the proper amount increases energy. Give the body time to adapt to the new changes and gently increase the demands. Patience is important here. It took awhile to get out of shape, didn't it? It'll take some time to get it back into shape as well. Patience and consistency are key. Once your body has adapted, it will be time to increase intensity levels.

Intensity Matters

Proper exercise intensity levels are critical to success. There is a balance to be achieved between not enough intensity and too much intensity. When the intensity is too low the body responds poorly which is physically ineffective and emotionally discouraging. When the intensity is too high the body responds poorly too, with increased fatigue and injuries, which can also be emotionally draining. There is a definite intensity sweet spot that is absolutely essential. Without it, failure and discouragement tend to prevail.

Let's look at low intensity issues. This is often a perception issue. Meaning that people think that they're putting in adequate work but they're not. I have to consciously stop my eyes from rolling when people tell me that they get plenty of exercise by "walking around at work" or by "chasing kids" all day. They act as though walking around or grabbing a toddler before they can get into things is something extraordinary for the body to handle. As compared to what? Do you suppose they really believe that their body was designed to sit all day instead, therefore the act of getting up, scooping up the child, or walking around your workplace is the formula for fitness? When people come to me and tell me that work or toddlers constitute plenty of exercise I promptly tell them, "obviously it is not," to which they promptly appear insulted. This goes back to a willingness to accept the truth, stop making up excuses, and take some personal responsibility. We're talking common sense here. If a person's so-called "toddler chasing" fitness regimen has not produced actual "fitness", then perhaps it's time to put it into proper perspective and call it "parenting" instead of "exercise".

Even when people put forth a more structured effort, if the intensity is inadequate, their effort will not be adequately rewarded. A prime example of this is *walking* as exercise. Walking is promoted as being one of the best forms of exercise. Walking has many benefits, primarily that it is cheap, easy, and convenient. Walking is an excellent place to start for someone who has been very sedentary. However, walking in itself is really not an exercise superstar. If you are an average person who is moderately active, then walking is probably not likely to produce a lot of physical changes. Think about it. You've been walking since you were about two years old. Why now would walking suddenly become so unique and intense to the body to produce a physical response from the body in terms of creating physical change for weight loss? You were designed to walk. You're supposed to walk! Again, for a very *sedentary* individual the act of participating in this very basic function of walking could produce some physical changes as the body begins to return to some level of *normal* function. For most everyone else, if you're going to walk, you had better walk *fast* or up some hills! In other words, you need to walk with *intensity* and effort...let's not forget duration. Walking is great exercise if it challenges you. Otherwise, your body is likely to treat it like a normal function that you were supposed to be doing anyway.

Walking combined with correct levels of intensity and duration can provide certain results. However as with all exercises, the type of exercise you choose determines the body's response which determines your overall results. Therefore, it is important to understand which types of exercises produce which types of outcomes. No matter which type you choose, you must exercise at a level which challenges the body to change. Without that challenge one can expect more of a "maintenance" response from the body, which is fine for some but not very useful for people trying to lose weight.

10,000 Steps? Maybe. I love pedometers and it's a pretty easy correlation to see that in general, the fewer the steps, the more likely the person will have a weight issue. Like everything else, the amount of steps needed is specific to the person, and some people have health conditions which disallow this step measurement to be useful. If you can safely walk, I think a pedometer is a great idea (one that is attached to you, not a phone app) because it encourages more *awareness*. Most people whom I work with initially tell me that they think they get "pretty close" to 10,000 steps… until I put an actual pedometer on them and they end up surprised that they are much lower than their perception.

If you use a pedometer as a tool, use it for a week and determine your average number of steps. Once you know your average, make that your minimum. By "minimum" I mean the number of steps you get no matter what! Each week, increase your minimum number by 200 steps, and listen for your body's feedback. This is an actual commitment here for this to work! Too little, your body will respond by NOT responding. Too much, your body will hurt. Just the right amount and your body will respond and feel good.

Do you need 10,000 steps? I don't know. Some people get positive feedback from their body with a 6000 step commitment. Mine insists upon 15,000 steps. Your body will tell you the right number.

Exercise Intensity and "Pain"

The intensity challenge is one of the hardest things for people to mentally overcome. People can actually experience a wide variety of emotions when exercise intensity levels increase to the point of discomfort or pain. The truth is that exercise has moments of physical discomfort and muscular burning (lactic acid) which is often perceived as pain. While joint pain should *never* be ignored and is a sign to stop, muscular "pain" is something that should be worked with.

Never try to ignore joint pain, even mild joint pain. If your knees, spine, shoulders, elbows, neck, wrists, hips, or ankles hurt…stop! Not all exercises are good for everybody. You have to see how *your* body is responding to it. Don't try to keep up with anyone else. You're building *your* healthy body, so only be concerned about *your* body's signals. If it's signaling pain, you need to heed the warning or you're likely to pay the price at some point. There's a big difference between joint and muscle "pain." Depending on your goals, a muscle that's "burning" is usually a good thing. That's a sign that your body has reached a response zone. However, even when those muscles are burning, you need to stop if your exercise technique begins to suffer so that you don't injure yourself. Herein presents the challenge.

When the exercise workload begins to get challenging that's when subconscious messaging can take over. A person with negative subconscious messaging may be having messages such as *"this is too hard"*, *"I can't do it"*, *"I'm embarrassing myself"*, *"I am weak"*, *"this hurts"*, *"I am out of shape"*, *"I can't keep up"*, *"I want to stop"*, *"I can't wait until this is over with"*, *"I give up"*. A person with positive subconscious messaging undergoing similar conditions may be having messages such as, *"I am determined"*, *"I am taking care of me"*, *"lactic acid is a good response"*, *"I am getting healthier"*, *"I can do it"*, *"I am determined to keep going"*.

The ability to handle physical intensity is directly associated to the subconscious mind's support and belief system of that intensity. Consciously the education has to be in place so that individual has the knowledge they need to understand the role intensity plays in achieving their desired physical outcome. Subconsciously that individual needs the support of positive internal messaging to help them work with the correct intensity to achieve their goals.

Affirmations that help are:
- ♥ "I am able to exercise intensely."
- ♥ "I am getting stronger all of the time."
- ♥ "I automatically respond to my body's needs by exercising to my true potential."

Am I willing to be patient and explore? The body de-trains at the approximate rate of 1% per day if a person becomes completely sedentary.

In other words you can't store fitness. Use it or lose it! Once you've lost it, it's going to take some time to get it back. Gradually increasing your fitness level is the smartest way to approach this lifestyle objective. Too much too soon will dramatically increase the dropout rate. Not enough will dramatically decrease the success rate. Finding that healthy balance of what works specifically for your body requires some patience and trial and error. It's about finding out what combination of activities work specifically for your body to help you achieve your specific goals.

Specificity in training means that you get what you do. Finding exercises that work for you and work with your personality are important for long-term adherence. Even intense exercise can be fun when you have found the style that appeals to you. Choose activities that you enjoy. This means you might have to experiment and try new things to discover what you like. Consider yourself an explorer! No matter how good a workout program may be, it simply won't work if you don't stick to it because you don't like it. Being fit and healthy gives you more opportunity to enjoy your life.

Affirmations that help are:
- ♥ "I am willing to try new exercises."
- ♥ "I enjoy trying new things."
- ♥ "My body is responding at the correct pace."
- ♥ "Every day that I exercise I get better and better."

Am I worth it? This is a bigger issue at stake here. If a person doesn't feel worthy it is unlikely that they will prioritize themselves enough to produce the commitment that is required for long term, lifelong health whether it is exercise or eating right. A person who doesn't value themselves appropriately is at high risk of being an exercise dropout. Most likely this person has a number of contributing factors when it comes to weight loss and emotional factors and internal perceptions need to be addressed in order to truly create change. If a person cannot answer this question (Am I worth it?) with a resounding *"yes"*, then there's little point in attempting to work with exercise intensity, mode, or frequency issues. Exercise is a head game. It starts there first. If your self-worth is low, work with that area. Exercise can help with confidence, but please take care of the bigger issue here. You matter.

Affirmations that help are:
- ♥ "I am worth it."
- ♥ "I am a priority."
- ♥ "I deserve to be healthy."

READ THIS AGAIN

Exercise burns calories, gives us more energy and helps us reduce our body fat percentage.

If what you are doing isn't working, that's a very strong indicator that your approach is not working well for your specific body and your specific goals.

Our bodies are uniquely coded and have needs based on that individuality.

Long term weight loss isn't a temporary goal, but rather it is a long term perspective change and application of healthy habits and behaviors as a lifestyle choice.

Proper exercise intensity levels are crucial to success.

Pay attention to joint pain, even mild joint pain.

Not all exercises are good for everybody.

The ability to handle physical intensity is directly associated to the subconscious mind's support and belief system of that intensity.

You can't store fitness. Use it or lose it.

Finding exercises that work for you and work with your personality are important for long-term adherence. This means you might have to experiment and try new things to discover what you like.

CHAPTER 13

THE WORKOUT PLAN

Much like "the diet" plan in chapter 11, the workout plan isn't set in stone either. The best "plan" is the one that is best for you, and it would be impossible for me to tell you what that is. Fortunately, you already have the answers, even if you don't realize it yet.

For starters, it's important to know some details about exercise so you can discover your answers more easily. Let's dive in, shall we?

Mode

Mode is the type of exercise that you participate in. For example: walking, kickboxing, weight training, yoga, dancing.

The mode affects results because of **specificity** of training. Specificity basically means *what you train for is what you get*. This is not the same thing as "spot reducing". There is no such thing as spot reducing... spot training, yes... spot reducing, no. Where our bodies like to collect body fat is mostly out of our control. The same is true for where our bodies shrink our fat cells. We can "spot tone" a body area, but we can't choose where our bodies lose fat. In other words, you can train your abdominal muscles to be toned and strong, but a layer of fat cells might still be sitting on top of your amazing abs, blocking the ability to visually see all of that hard work. This means that we have to know which modes (types) of exercises produce what types of responses in the body that we want.

The 5 Components of Fitness

The definition of physical fitness isn't a shape or weight. Physical fitness is the ability to physically be able to carry out the tasks that you need to and still have enough left over energy to do the things you want to. Still, there are elements that create a well balanced body in terms of fitness. These are the 5 components of physical fitness, which are flexibility, strength, endurance, cardiovascular fitness, and muscle vs. body fat ratios.

There are also 5 skill related components of fitness, which are balance, agility, power, speed, and coordination. For our purposes, we are going to focus on the physical components, although a well thought out approach also addresses the skill components, so do your best to factor them in.

Flexibility

Flexibility is the extensibility of the muscle. Flexible muscles can decrease pain, help with functional range of motion, and increase muscle efficiency. Stretching in itself is not a great "fat burning" activity, but because it helps the muscles to be more efficient, it helps the muscle cells uptake oxygen better which helps your cardiovascular workouts to be more effective for calorie burning.

There are different types of stretching with different goals. Rather than going into all of the details of that, I'll simply highlight a couple of rules:

- Warm up your muscles *before* doing mild, short (5-10 seconds) stretching before your workout, to prepare for the workout.
- After your workout, do longer (20 plus seconds), deeper stretching of the muscles used to recover from the workout and gain flexibility.
- Hold stretches (static) rather than bounce (ballistic) them.
- Stretching should feel like mild tension in the muscles, not pain.
- If your stretch makes your muscle shake, it's too intense. Back off a little bit.

Stretching doesn't have to be time consuming in order to give you benefits, it just has to happen. Even 5 minutes of your workout time can make an important difference. Having a couple of flexibility workouts, such as yoga, can be a great addition. However, preference, weekly time available, goals, and effectiveness might determine your stretching habits. Do include it though, even if it's a little.

Strength & Endurance

"Strength" is referring to how strong your muscles are. "Endurance" is referring to the stamina that your muscles have. Even if you don't care how strong your muscles are or how long they can work at any one time, muscle development and mass should be on your priority list for a number of reasons.

In terms of weight loss, the amount of muscle on your body influences your metabolism. More muscle equals a higher metabolism. Less muscle equals a lower metabolism. This means that we want muscle, because we will be better calorie burners!

As we age, if we are sedentary, we can lose up to 1% muscle mass per year! The loss in muscle mass can not only contribute to less joint stability, but increased annual weight gain. Muscle loss, along with the metabolic downshift that comes with it, makes losing weight and maintaining weight harder too!

From an aesthetic point of view, toned muscles are usually visually more appealing than soft muscles, and loose skin is less obvious as well when the muscles are genuinely firm.

Acquiring strong muscles doesn't mean that you have to become a gym rat or lift heavy weights. All it means is that you have to actively engage with your body's muscles 2-3 times per week to prompt a reaction from them.

There are different types of weight training or muscle conditioning according to your goals. Here are a few guidelines:

- "Overloading" a muscle means working it to exhaustion. This usually includes *lactic acid* build-up which causes that *burning* sensation that muscles can get when they are working hard.
- To gain muscle strength and size, overload a muscle using heavier weights with fewer repetitions. This is easier to accomplish with weight machines but can be done with minimal home workout gear

as well. How many times per week you should strength train depends on your goals and body type.

- To gain muscle endurance and tone, lift weights or do exercises where you can do several repetitions (20 and higher) before reaching muscle overload. This method tends to produce a leaner look to the muscles. Overload is still the goal though.
- For most women, it's hard to get "bigger" by working your muscles, but it's possible that certain body types might look leaner when they train their muscles more for endurance rather than strength. You will be able to see your changes in the mirror though, and it's easy to modify your approach. Bodies are moldable according to the exercises we choose.
- Burn baby burn! The discomfort that comes from muscular effort should be felt in the muscles, not the joints. If a joint hurts, STOP or modify the movement to alleviate the joint stress. If the muscle burns, give yourself a high-five.
- Warm up before using your muscles in this way.
- Work your opposing muscle groups in the same workout (biceps and triceps, back and abdominals, etc.).
- Do a variety of muscle conditioning exercises to avoid overuse issues and shape a healthier body.
- Be safe! Trust yourself. If it feels "wrong" it probably is.
- Personal trainers can be great assets, but so can fitness videos. Keep in mind that not every trainer or video will be right for you, and that's okay. Keep shopping if need be.
- Ask your doctor if there's anything you should or should not be doing regarding exercise, especially if you have a health issue or have had a previous injury.

Cardiovascular

Cardiovascular fitness is referring to the health and capacity of your heart and lungs. Aerobic exercise helps to train the heart and lungs to perform better. It's also important to know that it's an excellent way to burn fat.

When a person says they want to lose weight, what they usually mean is they want to burn excess storage fat on the body. Cardio workouts do just that!

So what is an effective cardio workout? It's any activity that elevates your heart rate and keeps it into a training zone for at least 20 minutes at a time. Yes, any activity will do. So if you hate treadmills, that's fine! How about dancing? Do you like exercise videos? Hiking? Biking? Heck, even cleaning your house could work if you do it in a hurry. Be creative, there are tons of options.

But remember, there are catches... the training zone and the time frame.

"THR" stands for Target Heart Rate. The training "zone" is where your heart rate needs to be in order to be in a training target heart rate zone. A target zone is a heart rate range that guides your workout by keeping your intensity level between an upper and lower heart rate limit. There are various target zones that are suggested for an individual to follow that correspond with a specific exercise goal. The general range for aerobic fitness is between 65% - 85%.

You gain the most benefits and lessen the risks when you exercise in your target heart rate zone. Usually this is when your exercise heart rate (pulse) is 65%-85% of your maximum heart rate. In some cases, your doctor may decrease your target heart rate zone to begin with 50%.

Decrease your exercise intensity if your heart rate during the activity exceeds your target heart rate. This increases both cardiovascular and orthopedic risk and does not add any extra benefit, unless you are training for a specific sport that requires it (like sprinting).

When beginning an exercise program, you may need to gradually build up to a level that is within your target heart rate zone, especially if you have not exercised regularly before. If the exercise feels too hard, slow down.

You will reduce your risk of injury and enjoy the exercise more if you don't try to over-do it!

The target rate zone is the best guess at measuring what energy system your body's using for your activity. This means a lot if you're trying to lose weight. Cardio workouts help the body burn fat, which means getting the body to use fat as a fuel source during exercise. The THR zone is the range in which the body recognizes the need to use extra fat to sustain your activity. Work out below the THR zone and your body probably won't change much (if any). Work out above the THR zone (anaerobic) and the body no longer uses fat as its fuel supplier, instead turning to glucose (sugars). Summary: The THR is the heart rate range that your body needs to be in to burn the most fat during exercise.

Before you can figure out what your training heart rate should be, you have to know what your resting heart rate is first. Your resting heart rate is the number of beats in one minute when you are at complete rest. Your resting heart rate indicates your basic fitness level. The more well-conditioned your body, the less effort and fewer beats per minute it takes your heart to pump blood to your body at rest. In other words, lower resting heart rates can be good indicators of cardiovascular fitness. As you become healthier, your resting heart rate should decrease. For this reason, you will want to re-calculate your resting heart rate every couple of months as you consistently exercise.

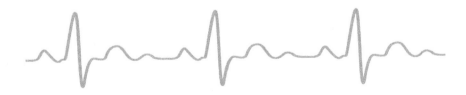

Getting Your Resting Heart Rate

✓ Wear a watch with a second hand.

✓ Either lie down & relax for 15 minutes with no stimulus (no reading, no TV, nobody talking to you, and so on). You can also do this first thing in the morning BEFORE getting out of bed (provided the alarm clock didn't scare you).

✓ Find your *pulse on your wrist or neck (don't press hard if you use your neck).

✓ Count your pulse for a full minute. If you lose count, start over. Don't guess.

✓ Write down your number.

✓ Repeat for three days in a row.

✓ Add the numbers up then divide your number by three to get your average. This number is your resting heart rate.

Not sure how to take your pulse? Place the tips of your middle finger and ring finger (third finger) on the palm side of your other wrist, below the base of the thumb. There is a groove between the inside wrist bone (radius) and the tendon below the base of your wrist. You can also lightly place the tips of your index and middle finger on your lower neck, on either side of your windpipe. However, if you use your right hand, test on the right side of your neck. If you use your left hand, test on the left side of your neck. Press lightly with your fingers until you feel the blood pulsing beneath your fingers. You may need to move your fingers around slightly up or down until you feel the pulsing. No matter which method you use, always use your fingers and not your thumb.

Now that you have your resting heart rate, it's time to determine your training heart rate zone.

Your Training Heart Rate

To get your training heart rate you will need to do a little math.

MEN:

220 minus your age = _____ (maximum heart rate)

Maximum heart rate (MHR) minus resting heart rate (RHR) = _____

X .65 + _____(resting heart rate) = _____Training Heart Rate (THR) @ 65%

220 minus your age = _____ (maximum heart rate)

Maximum heart rate (MHR) minus resting heart rate (RHR) = _____

X .85 + _____(resting heart rate) = _____Training Heart Rate (THR) @ 85%

Example: Bob is 45 and his resting heart rate is 72. The formula would look like this:

- ✓ 220 - 45 (age) = 175
- ✓ 175 – 72 (RHR) = 103
- ✓ 103 X .65 = 66.95
- ✓ 66.95 + 72 (RHR) = 138.95 (Round up to 139)

This means that Bob's training heart rate at 65% should be 139 beats per minute during cardiovascular exercise.

Do it again to determine what 85% should be.

- ✓ 220 - 45 (age) = 175
- ✓ 175 – 72 (RHR) = 103
- ✓ 103 X .85 = 87.55
- ✓ 87.55 + 72 (RHR) = 159.55 (Round up to 160)

This means that Bob's training heart rate at 85% should be 160 beats per minute during cardiovascular exercise.

Bob's training heart rate range should be between 139-160 beats per minute during cardiovascular exercise to be in a fat burning zone.

WOMEN:

226 minus your age = _____ (maximum heart rate)

Maximum heart rate (MHR) minus resting heart rate (RHR) = _____
X .65 + _____(resting heart rate) = _____Training Heart
Rate (THR) @ 65%

226 minus your age = _____ (maximum heart rate)

Maximum heart rate (MHR) minus resting heart rate (RHR) = _____
X .85 + _____(resting heart rate) = _____Training Heart
Rate (THR) @ 85%

Example: Angie is 52 and her resting heart rate is 60. The formula would look like this:

- ✓ 226 - 52 (age) = 174
- ✓ 174 – 60 (RHR) = 114
- ✓ 114 X .65 = 74.1
- ✓ 74.1 + 60 (RHR) = 134.1 (Round down to 134)

This means that Angie's training heart rate at 65% should be 134 beats per minute during cardiovascular exercise.

Do it again to determine what 85% should be.

- ✓ 226 - 52 (age) = 174
- ✓ 174 – 60 (RHR) = 114
- ✓ 114 X .85 = 96.9
- ✓ 96.9 + 60 (RHR) = 156.9 (Round up to 160)

This means that Angie's training heart rate at 85% should be 160 beats per minute during cardiovascular exercise.

Angie's training heart rate range should be between 134-160 beats per minute during cardiovascular exercise to be in a fat burning zone.

Remember, some people need to start out in a lower THR zone, particularly elderly, very sedentary people, or those who have or are recovering from certain health issues. It is always advised to consult with your medical doctor.

How to determine if you are in your THR range during exercise:

If doing a 10 second heart rate check (which means you stop to take your pulse for 10 seconds during a workout), divide THR by 6 to get range with a 10 second heart rate check. Repeat for both 65% & 85%.

Example: Angie's (from above) target THR is between 134-157.

134/6 = 22

157/6 = 26

Therefore if Angie takes her pulse for 10 seconds during activity, her goals would be to count 22-26 heartbeats during that 10 seconds.

If you are doing a 6 second heart rate check (which means you stop to take your pulse for 6 seconds during a workout), divide THR by 10 to get range with a 6 second heart rate check. Repeat for both 65% & 85%.

Example: Angie's target THR is between 134-157.

134/10 = 13

157/10 = 16

Therefore if Angie takes her pulse for 6 seconds during activity, her goals would be to count 13-16 heartbeats during that 6 seconds.

Other ways to monitor your workout.

If following "perceived exertion" or the "talk test": 65% feels like you are comfortably working, you could keep it up for a while, and you will be slightly winded. At 85%, you can definitely feel the heart & lungs working and you are breathing heavy (but not out of breath).

You're working out too hard (anaerobic) if you are breathless, gasping for air, or unable to easily speak a short sentence without taking a breath.

You're not working out hard enough if it feels "easy" and your breathing patterns have not obviously changed. If your heart & lungs are responding to your workout in a similar manner as if you were walking across a parking lot, or if you can easily talk in your regular speech patterns, you're probably not in the zone. Long time exercisers can fall into this easy zone as easily as anyone else, so it's a good thing to pay attention to it.

Muscle vs Body Fat Ratio

This is a measurement done to determine if you have the correct amount of body fat to muscle balance. This can be measured by a variety of methods including a bioimpedence machine, calipers, or underwater weighing. Whatever method you choose, you should re-check every 6 weeks or so and use the *exact* same method, including having the same person who initially measured this for you, if possible.

Body fat measurements and the measuring tape are wonderful methods for measuring weight loss, rather than relying on the scale. Remember, weight loss isn't really about losing weight, it's really about losing excess body fat. Understanding your body fat percentage helps you to realize the progress that is happening that the scale won't necessarily reflect.

First off, your body fat percentage is the percentage of fat your body contains. If you are 200 pounds and 30% fat, it means that your body consists of 60 pounds fat and 140 pounds of lean body mass (bone, muscle, organ tissue, blood and everything else). In this example, it doesn't mean losing 60 pounds is a goal. It means we need to know whether or not 30% is healthy or not.

A certain amount of fat is essential to bodily functions. Fat regulates body temperature, cushions and insulates organs and tissues and is the main form of the body's energy storage. Additionally, women need higher body fat percentages because of physiological differences such as hormones, ovulation, breasts, and sexual organs.

"Essential fat" is the minimum amount of fat necessary for basic physical and physiological health. Going below these numbers is <u>not</u> a goal.

"Athletic" is the category where there is visible muscle tone and definition throughout all or most of the body. These numbers should be watched closely, as people's bodies respond differently here. For example, one woman may look and feel fabulous at 15% body fat, while another woman at 15% body fat might experience hormonal issues because it's too low for her.

"Fitness" is typically the ideal, healthy range. Visually, this range produces a fit and healthy looking body without looking like you spend every spare minute in the gym. If you want to look "ripped", you need to be in the "essential" or "athletic" zone. Still, "fitness" zone looks great and is a healthy place for the internal workings of your body as well.

"Acceptable" is well... *acceptable*, although it's still considered a reasonable range in terms of health. In this range, you will see and feel a difference between the low and high numbers in this range. A person in the low range of "acceptable" can visually look toned while a person in the high range of "acceptable" can look softer (less toned). In this range you have minimized health risks to *average*. Think of it this way, the closer you are to the lower range the healthier you are. The closer you are to the higher range, the closer you are to fat associated health issues.

"Obese" is the category we want out of. Interestingly, the weight shown on the scale is not always a reflection of this zone. Visually thin people can measure as "obese". Remember, this is the measurement of the balance of body fat to the other tissues in the body. Skinny people can be obese. When a person is in this category it can be directly correlated with health outcomes. Obesity-related diseases include heart disease, type 2 diabetes, hypertension, and stroke. If you are in this category, this is a health and longevity concern.

After determining your body composition in terms of fat weight and lean weight, you can set a goal focused on positive and attainable objectives, such as losing 10% body weight or moving from one body fat classification category to the next.

Since lean mass can increase as a response to regular exercise, body composition re-assessments can help clarify if increases in weight numbers on the scale are a result of enhanced muscle or actual body fat. This can provide important information, especially when fat weight loss appears to have reached a plateau. Again, the scale alone can be misleading, which is why these other measurements can give a truer understanding of the body's response.

Remember to consider that "weight" consists of both lean body mass and body fat. Try to keep your weight loss goals realistic, and keep the calorie-burning muscle, and lose only the fat.

Conclusion

- ✓ Exercise. Exercise consistently using the correct modes, with the right amount of time and intensity.
- ✓ Re-evaluate your program and change it as your body gives you feedback. If your body is not responding, you need to change the approach. Your body is unique with its own unique requirements. You might have to experiment to find the combination that works for you.
- ✓ Cardio burns fat.
- ✓ Muscle building increases metabolism and helps you burn fat more efficiently.
- ✓ Flexibility training helps you burn fat more efficiently during your cardio workouts.
- ✓ Do it all (flexibility, cardio, and muscle work) to change body fat percentage ratios.
- ✓ Commit and prioritize. Your body needs you. Every. Single. Day.

READ THIS AGAIN

There is no such thing as spot reducing, only spot toning.

The THR is the heart rate range that your body needs to be in to burn the most fat during exercise.

Some people need to start at working out in a lower THR zone than others.

Your resting heart rate is the number of beats your heart beats in 1 minute while in complete rest.

Be safe! Trust yourself. If it feels "wrong" it probably is.

Ask your doctor if there's anything you should or should not be doing regarding exercise, especially if you have a health issue or have had a previous injury.

More muscle equals a higher metabolism.

CHAPTER 14

THE SCALE

To Weigh or Not to Weigh

It happens to all of us that own a scale. We hop on it, expecting to see good numbers as a reward for our recent good behaviors, and the scale betrays us! It taunts our efforts of exercising and eating salads! It's frustrating!

The scale can be a source of inspiration or discouragement, on any given day, with seemingly little rhyme or reason behind the numbers at times, and yet it remains a constant tool to measure whether or not we are fat, skinny, or just right. But is it accurate? Well, sort of.

For starters, you need to determine whether or not your scale is weighing correctly. Make sure that it's on a solid surface rather than carpet. If a digital scale has been recently moved, even an inch, it can throw its calibration off, so ignore the first reading if it was moved. To give your scale a quick test, weigh yourself 3 times in a row. You should get the same numbers. If not, try changing the batteries if applicable, or recalibrating. If you still get mismatched numbers, you probably need a new scale. Repeat this test with any new scale you purchase. Take it back for a refund if it doesn't pass your accuracy test. Just because it's new, doesn't make it better.

Once you have your properly working scale, either kick it off to the corner of your bathroom to be completely ignored or make a commitment to weigh every single day and record your weight. Hit-and-miss weigh-ins do not provide you with the information that you need. Unsystematic weighing tells you very little with anything less than 10 pound increments, and if you gain or lose 10 pounds, your clothes will point that out to you anyway. In other words, you don't need the scale to tell you whether you are gaining or losing. Now, if you are the type of person who really wants to weigh yourself, then fully commit, but understand *what* you are weighing first.

Technically, the scale is measuring your gravitational pull on Earth. It's measuring everything you put on it at one time…your clothes, your fat, your muscles, your hydration levels, your bones, your hair, your organs, undigested food …everything. Part of what it's weighing isn't even *you*! Ah ha! Does this explain the mystery of those wildly fluctuating numbers? Does this explain why one day you weigh one thing and the next day it's a few pounds higher or lower which may be in total conflict with what you thought it would be? Actually, yes.

Understand that the scale is weighing the whole package. If you are properly hydrated or dehydrated you will get a different number. If you have undigested food in your body, the scale is measuring that too, and you will get number fluctuations based on that. Obviously, external factors such as shoes and clothing will change numbers too. None of those things are actually you, and it's these types of factors that contribute to most random fluctuations, but we can minimize them by following these 3 steps.

Step 1: Weigh naked! (Okay, you can keep your socks on if you must, but naked is best).

Step 2: Weigh first thing in the morning…AFTER you pee…and BEFORE you eat or drink anything.

Step 3: Record your weight. Write it down or get an app for your phone to record it.

Why record it? Because you will STILL get fluctuations, but recording it helps you to better understand the difference between a normal fluctuation and actual weight gain or loss, as well as provide you with insight to some of your patterns. For example, if you notice that around the weekends your weight trends up, then that may indicate that there are some weekend choices that might be hindering you.

As far as understanding a fluctuation vs. a real change, here's how to do it:

1. Record your weight every day.
2. At the end of 7 days, add all the numbers up and divide by 7 to get your average weight.

WEEK ONE
Mon: 167.9
Tues: 166
Wed: 166.5
Thur: 163.5
Fri: 162.2
Sat: 167.4
Sun: 166.8
TOTAL: 1160.3
DIVIDE BY 7 DAYS

AVERAGE WEIGHT: 165.6

3. Repeat the next week.

WEEK TWO
Mon: 167.1
Tues: 166.3
Wed: 165.3
Thur: 163.5
Fri: 162.2
Sat: 163.4
Sun: 164.3
TOTAL: 1152.1
DIVIDE BY 7 DAYS

AVERAGE WEIGHT: 164.6

4. Now we have data to compare! Compare the differences between the week one average vs. the week two average.

Week 1: 165.6
Week 2: 164.6
WEIGHT DIFFERENCE: -1   A one pound weight loss!

By calculating averages, we are taking into consideration the fluctuations of hydration and digestion levels, which then gives us an overall more accurate picture of whether or not we are actually losing or gaining weight. If we just compared one day to another, it would be easy to be either falsely encouraged or discouraged, because it's far more likely for our numbers to be "off".

So now that we've cleared up some of the accuracy issues it's important to note that ideally, the scale is only *one* method that you use to monitor your progress, and it's still probably a great one. Because even when it's accurate as possible, it can still give you some confusing numbers as you get healthier. Yes, healthier.

As you incorporate more and more exercise into your lifestyle, your cells do a trade off of sorts. Muscle does *not* weigh more than fat (a pound of feathers weighs the same as a pound of bricks), but muscle is *more dense* than fat. In others words, a cubic inch of muscle will weigh more than a cubic inch of fat. For example, when I was at my fittest as an athlete fitness presenter, by body fat vs. muscle ratio percentage was in the high teens but I weighed 16 pounds more than I currently do! My body fat percentage is now in the low 20's, which is still healthy but now I have less muscle because I no longer exercise 14-20 hours per week. Also, I am close to the same size now as I was then... maybe a half size bigger now that I am 16 pounds lighter.

This muscle density increase and fat loss can create confusion on the scale! If we lose a pound of fat and gain a pound of muscle...according to the scale we made no progress, when we actually made tremendous

113

progress! By losing a pound of fat and gaining a pound of muscle we technically weigh the same but we've made some wonderful improvements for the body (increased metabolism, strength, endurance, energy, just to name a few). Additionally, your body will have *changed its shape,* which means that your clothes start fitting better and you start feeling better too. All of this, and the scale didn't even give you a high five.

With that said, it's also a good idea to check your physical measurements *and* have your body fat measured every 4-6 weeks or so, in order to have a more well-rounded outlook as to how your body is changing. Again, look at *trends* here and keep all measuring circumstances as similar as possible to better compare one set of numbers to the previous set.

To weigh or not to weigh? I say, either commit to the process of measuring *and* weighing or ignore it. Anything in between will probably be more confusing than helpful. Whatever you decide, remember there's always the easiest way to measure. Simply ask yourself a couple of questions:

How are your clothes fitting?
How are you feeling?

You can get these answers without any measuring devices at all...and sometimes it's those pure, honest answers that give you the most valuable information.

READ THIS AGAIN

The scale is measuring your clothes, your fat, your muscles, your hydration levels, your bones, your hair, your organs, undigested food...everything.

Muscle does not weigh more than fat (a pound of feathers weighs the same as a pound of bricks), but muscle is more dense than fat. A cubic inch of muscle will weigh more than a cubic inch of fat.

Either commit to the process of measuring and weighing or ignore it.

CHAPTER 15

OTHER INFLUENCING FACTORS

Sometimes, even when all of the right steps are consistently being taken, weight loss is harder than it should be, or a person will continue to gain weight. This is not to be confused with the fact that weight loss isn't an easy thing, or that true fat loss is slower than what the diet industry leads people to believe. I am talking about physiological reasons as to why things can be more difficult than expected for some people.

Some of these factors may require medical diagnosis and lab work to confirm. Some may even require intervention in the form of pharmaceutical medication or even surgery. The purpose of this chapter is not to diagnose, but to inform on some other factors that may need to be considered, as well as some natural health approach options.

Hypothyroidism

If your thyroid is underactive, your body may not produce enough thyroid hormone to help burn stored fat.

The thyroid is a small, butterfly-shaped gland that sits at the front of your neck. Your thyroid gland creates hormones that are responsible for a large number of bodily functions, including energy, body temperature, keeping organs functioning, and regulating metabolism. When thyroid hormone levels are low, people are more likely to gain weight because their body doesn't burn energy as efficiently as a body with a healthier thyroid.

The thyroid helps provide energy to nearly every organ in your body. Without the right amount of thyroid hormones, your body's natural functions begin to slow down.

Hypothyroidism affects women more frequently than men. It commonly affects people over the age of 60, but can begin at any age. Hypothyroidism is a fairly common condition, affecting around 10 million people in the United States. For most people, symptoms of the condition progress gradually over many years. As the thyroid slows more over time, the symptoms may become more obvious. Hypothyroidism can be diagnosed through a blood test, however "borderline" results that are still in the "healthy" range may still be impacting you. Taking symptoms into account can help you make good decisions in this area.

The signs and symptoms of hypothyroidism vary from person to person. The severity of the condition also affects which signs and symptoms appear and when. The symptoms are also sometimes difficult to identify as they can also be symptoms of other issues that are completely unrelated to your thyroid.

The most common signs and symptoms of hypothyroidism include:
- weight gain
- fatigue
- depression
- elevated blood cholesterol
- pain and stiffness in your joints
- dry, thinning hair
- constipation
- feeling cold
- dry skin
- muscle weakness, stiffness, aches, and tenderness
- decreased sweating
- slowed heart rate
- impaired memory
- fertility difficulties or menstrual changes
- hoarseness
- puffy, sensitive face

Hypothyroidism is often associated with an autoimmune disease. An example of that would be Hashimoto's disease. Hashimoto's disease is an autoimmune condition and the most common cause of an underactive thyroid. This disease attacks your thyroid gland and causes chronic thyroid inflammation. The inflammation can reduce thyroid function.

Other health issues can go along with hypothyroidism include celiac disease, diabetes, rheumatoid arthritis, lupus, adrenal gland disorders, pituitary problems, and sleep apnea.

Some people with hypothyroidism may only experience mood difficulties, leading to depression or anxiety. This can make diagnosing hypothyroidism or depression difficult, and can lead to the wrong treatment plan. Instead of only treating the brain, doctors should also consider testing for and treating an underactive thyroid. Depression is often a diagnosis made based on symptoms and medical history. Low thyroid function is diagnosed with a physical exam and blood tests. If the depression is caused only by hypothyroidism, correcting the hypothyroidism should treat the depression.

Blood tests are the best way to confirm a diagnosis of hypothyroidism. A thyroid-stimulating hormone (TSH) test measures how much TSH your pituitary gland is creating. If your thyroid isn't producing enough hormones, the pituitary gland will elevate TSH to increase thyroid hormone production. If you have hypothyroidism, your TSH levels are high, as your body is trying to stimulate more thyroid hormone activity. If you have hyperthyroidism, your TSH levels are low, as your body is trying to stop excessive thyroid hormone production.

A thyroxine level (T4) test is also very useful. T4 is one of the hormones directly produced by your thyroid. Together, T4 and TSH tests help evaluate thyroid function. Typically, if you have a low level of T4 along with a high level of TSH, you have hypothyroidism. However, there is a spectrum of thyroid disease, and additional thyroid function tests may be needed to properly diagnose your condition.

Medications for hypothyroidism
Hypothyroidism is usually medically treated by a synthetic version of the T4 hormone which copies the action of the thyroid hormone your body

would normally produce. The medication is designed to return adequate levels of thyroid hormone to your blood. Once hormone levels are restored, symptoms of the condition are likely to disappear or become more manageable

Alternative treatment for hypothyroidism
- Animal extracts that contain thyroid hormone are available. They contain both T4 and triiodothyronine (T3). One issue with the animal extracts is that they can be unreliable in dosing, so consistency and quality matter here.
- As a general rule, people with hypothyroidism don't have a specific diet they should follow. However, your thyroid needs adequate amounts of iodine in order to fully function. You don't need to take an iodine supplement in order for that to happen. A balanced diet of whole grains, beans, lean proteins, and colorful fruits and vegetables should provide enough iodine. Also, monitor soy intake. Soy may hinder the absorption of thyroid hormones.

Once you're treated for this condition, you may lose any weight that you've gained, because once your thyroid levels are restored your ability to manage your weight returns to normal.

Polycystic ovary syndrome (PCOS)
PCOS is a common condition that affects how a woman's ovaries work. The disease is a result of a hormonal imbalance and it affects more than 5 million women in the US. Symptoms can include irregular periods, acne, trouble getting pregnant, excess facial hair, thinning hair, and weight gain. The exact cause of PCOS is unknown, but it's thought to be hormone-related, including too much insulin and testosterone.

Cushing's Syndrome
Cushing's Syndrome is very rare, affecting around 1 in 50,000 people, and is caused by high levels of the stress hormone cortisol. When your body has too much of it, the excess hormone can throw off your body's other

systems. The condition, also known as hypercortisolism, is more common in women than men. It's most often seen in people ages 25 to 40.

You can get Cushing's syndrome when there's too much cortisol in your body for too long. Cortisol comes from your adrenal glands. It can develop as a side effect of long-term steroid treatment or as a result of a tumor. The most common cause is related to steroids. A tumor in your pituitary gland or a tumor in the adrenal glands, can also cause your body to make too much cortisol.

Weight gain is a common symptom, particularly on the chest, face, stomach, upper back, and base of the neck. It occurs because cortisol causes fat to be redistributed to these areas. Other symptoms can include rounded, rosy face, thinning skin, acne, fatigue, weak muscles, high blood pressure, depression, osteoporosis, kidney stones, sleep issues, hair growth on your body and face, irregular periods, irregular periods, and sexual issues.

Most cases of Cushing's syndrome can be cured. Depending on the cause, treatment typically involves either reducing or withdrawing the use of steroids, or surgery to remove the tumor.

Steroid Treatments

Steroids, also known as corticosteroids, are used to treat a variety of conditions. While this rarely leads to Cushing's Syndrome, long-term use of steroids seems to increase appetite and affects the areas in the brain that control feelings of hunger and fullness. In some people, this leads to weight gain. The higher the dose and the longer you are on steroids, the more weight you are likely to gain.

Syndrome X

Syndrome X is also known as insulin resistance or hyperinsulinemia. Syndrome X is a cluster of health conditions and is closely linked to obesity and inactivity. When your body is resistant to insulin, the other hormones that help your metabolism don't work as well.

Normally, your digestive system breaks down the foods you eat into sugar. Insulin helps sugar enter your cells to be used as fuel.

With insulin resistance, cells don't respond as they should and glucose can't enter the cells as easily. Because of this, your blood sugar levels rise as your body produces more and more insulin to try to lower your blood sugar.

Metabolic Syndrome

Metabolic syndrome is a cluster of issues that occur together, increasing your risk of heart disease, stroke and type 2 diabetes. These conditions include higher blood pressure, high blood sugar, extra body fat around the waist, and abnormal cholesterol or triglyceride levels. The more of these conditions you have, the higher your risk of complications, such as type 2 diabetes and heart disease.

Metabolic syndrome is common in the US, but serious and aggressive lifestyle changes can avoid and correct the issue.

Medications

Some medications can also cause you to gain weight or make it harder to lose it. Among the medications that may cause weight gain in some people are:

- Medications used to treat type 2 diabetes.
- Antipsychotic or schizophrenia medications.
- Beta-blockers.
- Antidepressants.
- Birth control pills.
- Hormone replacement therapy.
- Corticosteroids.
- Antiepileptics.

If you are gaining weight on a medication, your doctor may be able to help you find a similar drug that won't have the same effect. In some cases, there may be natural alternatives and options, but all changes in treatment options should be discussed with your doctor to ensure that it's safe for you to do so.

If you start a new medication, monitor your weight closely. If you see that you're gaining weight, tell your doctor so that adjustments can be made. As always, changing your diet and getting more exercise can also help, although it might take you longer than it otherwise would because of a medication.

Fatigue

Some studies have shown that people who get less sleep and are more likely to be overweight than those who get adequate sleep. One theory behind that dynamic is that sleep-deprived people have reduced levels of leptin, the chemical that makes you feel full, and higher levels of ghrelin, the hunger-stimulating hormone. Additionally, if you're always feeling tired, you are more likely to reach for high-calorie and sugary snacks to try to keep your energy levels up throughout the day. You are also more likely to turn to convenience foods and less likely to engage in physical activity, all of which add up to weight gain.

Unhealthy Relationships

Our relationships have direct impact on our emotions and happiness and can impact food and exercise behaviors. I've seen many cases where one person will sabotage the other's success, or try to make things difficult. In some cases, a person is actually trying to be helpful, but their words hurt and make things worse. If you have someone who is toxic to your health, discuss with them exactly what you need from them. If they aren't willing to have that talk and try to meet your needs, you may have bigger decisions to make regarding that relationship.

Age & Hormones

People naturally begin to lose modest amounts of muscle as they get older because they tend to become less active, but hormone changes factor in as well. Changes in hormonal levels can accelerate muscle loss. While hormonal downshifting is normal, if it begins to interfere with quality of life, there are natural solutions that can help the body to age a bit more gracefully with fewer side effects.

Muscles are efficient calorie burners, so a loss of muscle mass can mean you are burning fewer calories. This muscle loss also affects the metabolism and how much energy the body burns at rest. Basic organ function accounts for about 70 percent of metabolic rate. Most of the remainder comes from maintenance of lean muscle tissue. Fat burns very little calories at rest. People with lower amounts of muscle tissue do not burn as many calories at rest as someone with more muscle, making weight loss more difficult. Older adults tend to have less muscle and a lower base metabolism.

In other words, even if you are eating and drinking the same amount as you always have, as you age, you are more likely to gain weight. To reduce muscle loss, you should stay active and try to do regular muscle conditioning exercises, with an ultimate goal of gaining muscle. Having more muscle will help control weight, increase energy levels, improve stamina, support joints, and lead to a higher quality of life.

Chronic Stress

When you live with ongoing anxiety or stress, your body can produce chemical substances, like the hormone cortisol, that make your body more likely to store fat, especially around the waist. There may also be a tendency to eat due to emotions, rather than legitimate hunger.

Stress is a normal part of life, so this does not mean that weight issues are a given. It simply means to pay attention to your emotions and stress levels. If it feels ongoing and overwhelming, it's time to develop some skills and strategies to cope. You can simultaneously become emotionally stronger while you are getting your body physically stronger.

Everything is connected. To be the healthiest you, you have to look at your emotional well-being as well.

Drinking the Weight

- **Alcohol** in moderate to excessive amounts can sabotage your efforts to lose weight. Alcohol (including beer and wine) is a refined carbohydrate, similar to sugar. Besides adding calories, alcohol may raise blood sugar and insulin levels, which can contribute to weight gain.
- **Fruit juice**, while having nutritional value, is calorie dense. Rather than going for the juice, go for the actual fruit instead. This doesn't mean that unsweetened juice is "bad," it just means that you need to be aware of your choices.
- **Fancy Coffee Drinks.** Black coffee has zero calories, but many coffee shop drinks are calorie bombs and can contain more calories than a hamburger and fries! Take the time to learn the nutritional content in food and drinks before consuming them.
- **Smoothies.** Again, you might be drinking the caloric equivalent of a meal or two here. If your intention was to substitute a meal, that's one thing. But if it wasn't, it could be a problem. So again, understand the nutritional and caloric meaning before assuming it's healthy or a good choice, especially if it's a smoothie that you order rather than make at home.

Many people easily lose weight by giving up all of the extra calories of unnecessary beverages. Go for zero to low calorie drinks, pure water being the champion choice.

What about diet drinks?

This may come as a surprise if you are used to diet dictatorship, but having a diet drink or soda is not really a big deal for most people. There have been stories out there in the land of the internet that claim that diet soda causes weight gain, so it's healthier to choose the real sugar over the artificial sweetener. Ummmm, I hate to be Captain Obvious here, but the body needs calories in excess to gain weight. Zero calorie drinks are.... ZERO calories. It's impossible to gain weight as a result of drinking zero calories. Those who claim that the artificially sweet taste causes sugar cravings, actually have issues with "cravings" which are not actually the result of the diet soda. I know some people who say that a diet soda can help them to satisfy a sweet craving, not cause one. I suppose that part would be up to your individual experience.

I know professional fitness competitors that drink excessive diet sodas every day and they are lean as can be. Now, this does not mean that I think drinking a ton of diet drinks are a good or healthy choice. Artificial sweeteners can indeed be problematic and one really should heed some caution when choosing the type of sugar replacement as well as the amount and frequency. It's also good to note that some people are sensitive to sugar alternatives and get side effects, headaches being one of the most common.

The healthiest choice? Water of course, preferably purified in some manner. If choosing to drink teas or coffee, try them without sweeteners. If you really need some sweetness, look into natural sources such as stevia or monk fruit.

Caffeine

Some people are sensitive to caffeine and are better off reducing or eliminating it. Since caffeine acts as a de-hydrant, it can also negatively impact the hydration level of your body which can make weight loss harder because you want your body to be fully hydrated for the best results. So if there are no other fluid sources besides caffeinated beverages, this can be a real problem. However, there are some benefits with regards to weight loss to drinking caffeine in moderate amounts.

Caffeine mixed with healthy carbohydrates can replenish the glycogen in your muscles up to 66% faster after exercise. Caffeine can also lessen oxidative stress on the joints and muscles and diminish inflammatory responses during endurance activities. Caffeine increases stamina during exercise and can relieve post-workout muscle pain by up to 48%.

Research from a German study showed that weight loss study participants who drank 2-4 cups of coffee a day were more likely to be successful at keeping the weight off than those who did not drink caffeine.

Now before you run out and order that cup of coffee, notice that it helped because of the exercise factors, and it's also talking about 2-4 cups of plain coffee. There's a method to it. Too much caffeine can have negative results.

Dog Ownership

According to the American Heart Association, owning a pet, particularly a dog, decreases the risk of obesity. Dogs should be walked daily and are often quite persistent, encouraging their owners to walk as well. Young dogs and active breeds also have play needs which a good pet owner will respond to. This equates to more calories burned by spending some extra time with that hairy buddy. Besides, research shows that petting an animal greatly reduces stress and depression, two other known risk factors for weight gain. So if you do have a dog, take them for a walk and enjoy all of those snuggles.

Money

Income *can* be correlated with obesity, with poor Americans being more likely to be obese than richer ones. Low-income people are less likely to purchase fresh foods, less likely to have health insurance, less likely to have gym memberships, and less likely to live in neighborhoods where exercise outdoors is encouraged or even safe. People with money can afford high quality foods, gyms, doctors, and personal trainers. Low income populations tend to choose more "dollar menu" items and low quality grocery items such as Ramen and other processed foods. When produce is an option, organic produce is often overlooked because of the price differences with the non-organic counterparts. That too, can create a problem.

It is important to note that a person *can* exercise and eat well on a tight budget. The money correlation is merely a generalization, not a determining factor of outcome.

Pesticides

Regular exposure to pesticides through food was correlated with an increase risk of obesity. Pesticides may help grow stronger and more abundant crops but many of the chemicals used are known "endocrine disruptors", meaning that they can interfere with your body's metabolic systems. Pesticides can disrupt our metabolism by interfering with the body's natural hormones. Buying all organic and non-GMO, as well as drinking filtered or reverse osmosis water can help, but for many people that doesn't fit in the budget. If money's tight you can also decrease your pesticide exposure by avoiding, or only buying organic of the most contaminated produce. The most contaminated are usually the produce with nooks and crannies, such as broccoli or strawberries. I save money by purchasing non-organic produce that has a peel that I am not going to eat, like bananas. However, if I am going to eat the outer layer or the whole thing, like a bell pepper or lettuce, I always buy organic. Another great option is to grow your own organic produce, but when purchasing seeds or seedlings, make sure you are getting organic and non-GMO seeds or plants to start out with, and use untreated dirt. Also, there are plenty of options for organic, non-dangerous pest control. You may just have to do a little research and experimenting, but it will be worth it. Organic garden produce tastes amazing compared to the chemical experiments disguised as produce found in the average grocery store.

READ THIS AGAIN

Everything is connected.

CHAPTER 16

SELF ASSESSMENT

How many things do you need to address in order to rebalance your thoughts, your beliefs, and your habits in order to achieve your healthiest self and create a connected relationship with your body?

Let's look at things from a different angle now and turn the attention to self reflection. Stay objective and be utterly honest. After all, this is your book. Use it as a tool to help you get to where you want to be, and perhaps discover the ways to get there. Taking a personal inventory helps to determine what areas may need attention.

Check off which statements currently apply to you. If you are unsure, put a question mark by it.

_____ Food is in control.
_____ I can't say "No" to food and mean it.
_____ My portions are too big.
_____ My portions are too small.
_____ I am not really sure what correct portions are.
_____ I binge eat (gorging).
_____ I binge drink.
_____ If I binge, I make myself throw up.
_____ I eat differently in secret.
_____ I do not eat enough fruits (1-2 servings) and vegetables (3-7 servings)
_____ I do not eat the right amount of protein.
_____ I am not really sure what the right amount of protein is.
_____ I do not eat the right amount of complex carbohydrates.
_____ I am not really sure what the right amount of complex carbohydrates are.
_____ I eat too many simple carbohydrates.

_____ I am not really sure what the difference is between simple and complex carbohydrates.

_____ I eat too much fat.

_____ I am not really sure about how much fat I should be eating.

_____ I think about food all of the time.

_____ My thoughts about food can feel obsessive.

_____ My thoughts about my weight and my body feel obsessive.

_____ Food feels like an "addiction" to me.

_____ I eat for reasons that have nothing to do with hunger.

_____ I eat when I am feeling emotional (stressed, mad, sad, lonely, etc.).

_____ I use food as an emotional distraction.

_____ I eat when I am bored.

_____ I eat late at night or right before bed.

_____ I eat out often.

_____ When I am at a restaurant, I make unhealthy choices.

_____ I do not plan any of my meals in advance.

_____ I do not make sure that healthy foods are available to me.

_____ I can't tell when I am full.

_____ I can only tell if I am full if I am "stuffed".

_____ I do not stop eating when I am full.

_____ I eat fast.

_____ I overeat due to taste.

_____ I do not usually leave food on my plate, even if I am full. I clear my plate.

_____ I skip meals.

_____ I don't get enough sleep.

_____ I snack between meals, even if I am not hungry.

_____ I have uncontrollable food cravings.

_____ I crave sugar.

_____ I crave salty foods.

_____ I crave high fat foods.

_____ I have fears about losing weight.

_____ I use weight as a form of protection.

_____ I do not exercise enough.

_____ I am not sure what the right amount of exercise is.

_____ I do not exercise consistently.

_____ I do not exercise with the correct intensity for my goals.

____ I am not sure what the right amount of exercise intensity is right for me.

____ I hate exercise.

____ I won't make time to exercise.

____ I am not motivated to exercise.

____ I do not drink enough water.

____ I am not sure how many ounces of water my body needs to function well and lose weight.

____ I drink sugary drinks.

____ I consume alcohol.

____ I drink excessive amounts of caffeine.

____ I do not appreciate and respect my body.

____ I hate my body.

____ My relationship with my body is terrible.

____ I don't understand my body.

____ I do not understand how to listen to my body.

____ My "self-talk" is mostly critical.

____ I have issues with judgment and/or I think people judge me because of my weight.

____ Other people can affect my weight or how I feel about my body.

____ I sabotage my own efforts.

____ I have someone in my life that sabotages me or makes me feel unsupported.

____ I have weight-related parental issues.

____ My over-all confidence is generally low.

____ I do not feel worthy. My self-worth is low.

____ My self-esteem is low.

____ I take care of others, but do not take care of myself.

____ I am not a priority.

____ I am confused about which diet to follow.

____ I can't get the diet mentality out of my head.

____ Food feels like an addiction.

____ I use food as a reward.

____ I use food or weight as self-punishment.

____ I am not motivated to change how I eat.

____ I am not confident that I can lose weight or maintain weight loss.

____ I think I am too old to lose weight.

_____ I want my body to change quickly, no matter the cost.

_____ I am unsure what reasonable expectations and pace are for my body to lose weight in a healthy manner.

_____ I have a health, hormonal, or medication issue that affects my weight.

_____ I may possibly have a health, hormonal, or medication issue that affects my weight, but I am not sure.

_____ Other_____

_____ Other_____

_____ Other_____

This list should help you to identify the areas that need attention. Any box that is checked off is potentially having a negative impact on your weight and health. Don't freak out if there's a lot of things checked off. This is merely information gathering to help you identify areas that may be affecting you that you might not have considered before. Later we will use this information to chart progress. For now, explore these areas more, look at what they might mean, and what to do about it.

Looking Closer

_____"Food is in control" _or_ "I can't say "No" to food and mean it." _You are a thinking, strong, intellectual being, food is not. Food is necessary for survival, but it should never be given authority over how you eat, as food is not the intelligent being, you are._

_____"My portions are too big" or "My portions are too small" or "I am not really sure what correct portions are." _Let your body guide you. Eat when you are hungry and stop when you are full. Do your best to pay attention. As you practice this, it will become easier to recognize your body's signals._

_____"I binge eat" or "I binge drink" or "If I binge, I make myself throw up." _Obviously, all of this indicates an out of control relationship with food or alcohol that is clearly unhealthy. If you binge, spend some time reflecting upon why it happens. Notice if there are triggers and address the triggers. Talk to a_

132

professional if needed, which is usually a good course of action, as this can lead to other health issues.

___**"I eat differently in secret"** *The relationship you have with your body is between you and you. Your choices should match whether you are eating alone or with others. If not, examine more closely why that is. It could give you another clue as to what changes should be made.*

___**"I do not eat enough fruits (1-2 servings) and vegetables (3-7 servings."** *The healthiest diets in the world are plant based. I am not trying to convince you to be a vegetarian, but plants are nutrient rich, low calorie, and contain enzymes. People almost always look and feel better when they are consuming enough produce. If loving produce doesn't come natural to you, perhaps you might benefit from exploring different types and preparation methods. Also, it doesn't have to be complicated. Fresh is best, but if frozen works better for you then go for it! Even canned vegetables are better than none. This has to work with your style to work.*

___**"I do not eat the right amount of protein"** or **"I am not really sure what the right amount of protein is"** *Re-read chapter 9. Typically, most people need around 3 oz of protein per meal (about the size of a deck of cards), but protein needs vary according to goals, medical issues, and exercise levels.*

___**"I do not eat the right amount of complex carbohydrates"** or **"I am not really sure what the right amount of complex carbohydrates are."** *Re-read chapter 9. Complex carbohydrate needs vary according to goals, medical issues, and exercise levels. Remember, these are the good carbs! Your body and your brain need them.*

___**"I eat too many simple carbohydrates"** or **"I am not really sure what the difference is between simple and complex carbohydrates are."** *Re-read chapter 9. It is important to have these differences memorized.*

___**"I eat too much fat"** or **"I am not really sure about how much fat I should be eating."** *Re-read chapter 9. For weight loss, limit fats to less than 45 grams per day. Less than 30 grams a day would be even better.*

___**"I think about food all of the time"** or **"My thoughts about food can feel obsessive"** or **"My thoughts about my weight and body feel** obsessive" or **"Food feels like an "addiction" to me."** *Being <u>aware</u> is very different than obsessing. Once you stop the diet cycle and start looking at food logically, most obsessive thoughts will go away. Once you understand your body better, you can develop reasonable expectations and stop the internal pressure you have put upon yourself. It's okay to be <u>aware</u> that your body is in progress. If thoughts feel obsessive, try practicing re-directed self-talk (chapter 5) to change the thoughts or even to shut them off.*

___**"I eat for reasons that have nothing to do with hunger"** or "**I eat when I am feeling emotional** (examples: stressed, mad, sad, lonely" or "**I use food as an emotional distraction"** or **"I eat when I am bored."** *If you truly begin to eat only if your body is actually hungry, your body will begin to regulate your weight as to what you need, with very few exceptions.*

If you eat when you are bored, write a list of alternate things you can do when you are bored. Include project and chores, but also fun things and hobbies. Include time consuming things as well as things that just take a few minutes and everything in between. Write this list down and put it on your fridge. If you find you have wandered into your kitchen out of boredom, defer to your list instead. Another trick I do is to have a bowl of apples and oranges on the counter. If I am not sure if I am hungry, I ask myself if I want to eat the apple. If the answer is "No, I am looking for something else", it's a quick clue that actual hunger is not actually driving my decisions, and it's time to re-direct.

If you eat for comfort or emotional reasons, it's probably time to take a closer look at those emotions. Remember, food is just a substance that has nothing to do with stress, anger, or any other emotion. So instead of ignoring why you are feeling an emotion by attempting to create a mental diversion with food, take a closer look at the emotion <u>and</u> the cause. If you address the cause, you may find yourself solving some problems that need solving. Even if it's nothing you can fix, you still have the option of ignoring it if you want to. Either way, it still has nothing to do with food.

If stress and emotions cause you to eat, it's time to take control. Sit down and work out a mini stress-management program which answers the following questions:

- ***What are the situations, emotions, or people that cause you to stress eat?*** *Anger, frustration, boredom, the boss, etc.*
- ***How can you deal with these situations and emotions without eating?*** *Example: If you eat while driving, have less fattening nibbles at hand.*

Example: If a friend or relative forces you to eat platefuls of fattening food each time you visit, fill up before you visit and decline her cooking (or just have a few bites).

- **Can you avoid these situations?**
  Example: If you always eat junk in front of the TV, then watch less TV!
  Example: If seeing Mr. X makes you stress eat, consider avoiding him.

- **What tools can help you relieve your stress?** *Exercise is an excellent stress reliever, so is talking with a friend, meditation, hypnosis, yoga, and a multitude of other productive choices. Find what works for you.*

Stress and emotional eating can be triggered by complex issues. The message here is to learn to recognize what the issue or trigger is, so you can problem solve and move past it. In a nutshell - TAKE CONTROL! Don't allow people or situations to cause you to gain weight. Think about your situation and solutions in advance.

___**"I eat late at night or right before bed."** *Providing calories right before bed means that you are dumping calories into the body at a time when your body is the slowest at burning calories. If it's late and you are genuinely hungry, and assuming you will ultimately be in a reasonable calorie range for the day, try to eat the minimum amount to satisfy the hunger. Another indicator of eating too much to close to bed is whether or not you are hungry in the morning. If you are not, it's a good indication that your body is still working on the food from the previous night. Hunger in the morning is a good sign. Obviously, if you work an unusual schedule you would adjust everything according to your sleep and rise times.*

___**"I eat out often."** *It's much easier to control your fat intake and food quality when you prepare it yourself, not to mention much more cost effective.*

___**"When I am at a restaurant, I make unhealthy choices."** *Portion sizes are usually too big at restaurants and there are plenty of unhealthy choices on most menus. However, there are usually a few healthy options (besides ordering a salad). If you listen to your body's satiety signals and stop eating when you are full, then you will usually eat the right amount. Have the leftovers boxed up to take home or if you don't trust yourself, ask the server to remove your plate. Have an inattentive server? Put your used napkin in the plate and push it away. Another approach is to ask the server if they offer half or smaller portions. Many restaurants do, even if it's not listed on the menu.*

If you make poor choices because you are socializing or feeling food pressures, you may need to remind yourself that your body is your business, completely separate from what somebody else wants to order. This may require some self reflection to think about why this dynamic affects you.

Then there are the dreaded buffets... where people like to eat their money's worth. Buffets are usually quite high fat, as the restaurant has a financial motivation to use fat as a filler. One smart tactic is to make your first plate a "sampler"plate. Get a tablespoon or so of each item you are interested in. When tasting your sampler plate, try a small bite first. If you don't like it, don't finish it (that way you don't feel guilty about the food waste, if that's an issue). Once you have finished your sample plate, you might be full so you are simply done. If you are still hungry, go back and get more of the things you enjoyed. As always, stop when you are full. Yes, it's a good idea to avoid fried foods, creamy foods, cheesy foods, sugary foods, or basically anything that looks like it's swimming in an oil spill. But this isn't an exercise in deprivation; it's an exercise of strategy that balances taste preferences with intelligence to avoid gluttony.

When all else fails, simply eat out less. There are plenty of meal delivery services out there that make food shopping and preparation easier than ever before. Use the tools that make your success easier.

____**"I do not plan any of my meals in advance."** *Meal planning just makes things easier. I am not talking about planning every single meal (that might make you crazy), but at least plan your main meal. Here are the basics of meal planning:*

1. **Determine how many days your plan is for.** An easy way to decide this is to determine how many days are in between grocery store trips. For example, if you shop on the same day every week, once a week, then your plan should be for 7 days. If your schedule allows you to shop every 3 days, then your plan only needs to be for 3 days. Shopping for longer stretches (past 7 days) might not be as productive as your fresh produce may start to wilt or over ripen, which could create more waste.

2. **Determine what meals your plan covers.** Some people prefer to only plan the trickier meals (like dinner), while some people do better planning every meal. Whichever method you use, just make sure you end up with good food choices available to you. Just because you "plan" for a snack doesn't mean you have to eat it (if

you are not hungry then you obviously don't need it). However, if you need a snack, it's good to be prepared and have healthy choices readily on hand.

3. **Keep balance in mind.** Change meat options and include vegetarian meals. Create balance by making sure you are having complex carbohydrates, protein, and plenty of veggies.

4. **Grab your cookbook or other healthy recipe source, a pen, and paper to write your list on.** Give yourself a resource to find recipes and start looking for meals that peak your interest. Attaching your paper to a clipboard while you write can also be nice to use, not only for making your plan and grocery list, but it will be easier to have a firm surface to work with while you are crossing things off your list while you are at the store.

5. **Fill out your meal plan and make your grocery list as you are choosing your meals.** For example, if you want to eat oatmeal and blueberries for breakfast, then you need to add oatmeal and blueberries to your grocery list.

6. **Organize your grocery lists according to the aisle that you are likely to find the food in.** Make actual headings like "produce", "dairy", "meat", etc. It makes it much faster when it's time to shop, and keeps you from wandering the junk aisle.

7. **Write down everything you might potentially need for your plan to be followed.** This includes things like spices. This may seem like extra writing, but it will keep you in "planning" mode if you are not disrupting yourself by constantly checking your cabinets while you are trying to make your list.

8. **Check your stock-up list and add to your grocery list.** Keep a mini list on your fridge for incidentals as you run out of them. Then when you are ready to go to the store, simply transfer the mini-list to your master list. This keeps you from not having spices, and common ingredients on hand, as well as non-food items, like dish soap. If you live with others, ask them to write down items on the stock-up list if they use the last of an item. If they used all of the eggs, they simply write eggs on the list, so you know to add eggs to your master grocery list.

9. **Shop your own pantry, fridge, and freezer before going to the store.** Now that you made your list, see if you already have some of

those items. There's no point in buying more chicken if you already have chicken in the freezer that needs to be used up.

10. **Once you are at the store, only purchase what is on your list.** This will keep you from randomly grabbing things (which runs up your food bill). Plus, if you leave the junk food at the store (because it's not on your list), you've already eliminated most of the temptation. Saying no to the cookies that are in the grocery store is easier than saying no to the cookies sitting in your kitchen. Think about it.

___**"I do not make sure that healthy foods are available to me."** *Re-read the previous section on meal planning. If you plan for success, it's far easier to be successful.*

___**"I can't tell when I am full."** *Slow down and really start to pay attention. Try letting yourself get a little hungry (not ravenous). Eat slowly. Eat until you notice that the hunger went away. Don't worry, you can eat more later if you get hungry again. Tuning into your body is a wonderful way to connect to it and let it start guiding you. Sometimes your mind and body have to be re-trained in this area because a person has ignored it for so long. If that's you, it will re-learn, and you will start getting signals.*

___**"I can only tell if I am full if I am "stuffed".** *You are probably eating too fast and without being aware. Slow down and pay attention. Read on.*

___**"I do not stop eating when I am full."** *Why is that? Really. Ask yourself that question. This could mean many things, most of those things are in this list somewhere. Take the time to give yourself an answer.*

__**"I eat fast."** *The easy answer is to slow down. There are a lot of tricks people use... chewing their food a certain number of time, putting the fork down between bites, drinking water before each bite, etc. However, eating fast only really becomes a weight issue if it causes overeating. Some of you might have jobs or situations where leisurely eating isn't always an option, so you don't need to feel bad if you eat a fast meal. If you have pre-portioned your lunch and you are consuming 500 calories, it's not terribly relevant whether or not it takes you 3 minutes or 30 minutes to eat it. Granted, your digestive system will appreciate it more if you eat slower and properly chew your foods... but 500 calories is still 500 calories, no matter how fast they went in. However, if your meal isn't* proportioned, it's very hard to get a "stop eating" signal before it's too late and you have eaten too much. Slow down when you can. Pre-portion when you can not.

___**"I overeat due to taste."** *Hey, I love food too. Food is awesome! I get that it's tempting to eat a little more because it tastes good. But ask yourself if you are willing to give some extra exercise time for those extra bites. Be honest. You can trade like that. But you can't expect your body to become lean if you intake more than you outtake. Here's another thought; if it tastes so great, save some for later so you can enjoy it two times instead of once! Afraid that someone will eat your fabulous leftovers? Disguise them in some non-transparent container and put them in the back of the fridge or cupboard. You are clever, you will think of something. Now, this is not the same thing as hiding food to eat in secret. You are merely effectively reserving your uneaten portion of healthy, delicious food, so you can have more later when your body is hungry again, while protecting your food from fridge raiders.*

Seriously though, taste should be enjoyed. Overeating causes issues that are not enjoyable. Heart disease doesn't taste good. Keep your eye on the big picture.

___**"I do not usually leave food on my plate, even if I am full. I clear my plate."** *Having the need to clear your plate is often a remnant from what we were taught as children. I grew up this way, so I would eat all the food off of my plate in order to have seconds of what I liked. I carried this bad habit into adulthood and it would cause me to overeat. I had to un-do that childhood training and remind the adult me that I do not have to eat every bit of food on my plate in order to have seconds of what I wanted. I also had to let go of the guilt of wasting food, if I scraped unwanted food into the garbage. I still like to try new foods that I haven't tried before, and that can be fun. But I certainly won't continue to eat it if I don't like it. Just as important is the ability to stop eating as soon as you are full, even if there are only a few bites left. I have met many women who even eat the leftovers from their kid's or husband's plate. The rule of thumb here is simple… if you are no longer hungry or don't like it, stop eating. Throw the leftovers away or store them for later. Still think it's wasteful to throw away those few bites on your plate? You are right! You will be <u>wasting your time</u> and <u>wasting your effort</u> towards your weight loss goals. If it bothers you that much, store those few bites as leftovers. Silly to dirty a dish to store those few bites in? Would you rather spend a minute washing a dirty food storage container after it stored a few bites you will probably never eat, or would you rather spend a larger* *amount of time exercising off the extra calories that those few bites were composed of? Think about it. It's all about choices.*

___**"I skip meals."** *Breakfast tends to be the most commonly skipped meal, but certainly others get ignored or avoided. Skipping meals can cause a downshift in metabolism, as the body will slow down the rate in which it burns calories if the tank is empty, so to speak. This is not to suggest that you eat a meal if you are not hungry, but to evaluate why you are skipping it. If you are not hungry, is it because you ate too much earlier? If you are skipping breakfast, is it because you ate too late the night before? Do you skip meals because you don't have time? If that's the case, remember that it's not actually having a "meal" that wakes up your metabolism, it's just calories. It could be as simple as grabbing a banana and eating it on your way to work. I always keep a box of protein bars in my desk at work, that way if I don't have time for a proper lunch, I at least have a protein bar as a back-up plan.*

___**"I don't get enough sleep."** *A study in the journal "Sleep" found that people who were sleep-deprived were less able to resist cravings, This resulted in weight gain. Insufficient sleep is correlated to increases in hunger and food intake which exceeds energy demands of extended wakefulness. Endocannabinoids are naturally synthesized lipids that bind activate receptors that promote hedonic eating. When a person gets adequate sleep, blood levels of the most abundant endocannabinoid increase from mid-sleep to early afternoon. With sleep restriction, the endocannabinoid level is increased, coinciding with greater desire for food. Additionally, sleep deprivation can trigger sugar cravings.*

Lack of sleep also affects our ability to lose weight because it affects hormones. The two hormones that are key are ghrelin and leptin. Ghrelin is the 'go' hormone that tells you when to eat, and when you are sleep-deprived, you produce more ghrelin. Leptin is the hormone that tells you to stop eating. When you are sleep deprived, you have less leptin. It all adds up to more ghrelin plus less leptin equals weight gain.

Seek out sleep solutions. Natural choices can help you get your needed rest and put an end to the cycle. Some of those include:
- ⌘ *Passion Flower: Provides a calming effect to support relaxation.*
- ⌘ *Melatonin: Maintains normal sleep cycles. 3 mg works best for most people.*
- ⌘ *L-Theanine: Supports relaxation.*
- ⌘ *Valerian Root: Supports muscle relaxation.*

⌘ *CBD/CBG: Anxiety, sleep, and pain. Formulas vary a great deal, so do some research to see what is best for you.*

___**"I snack between meals, even if I am not hungry."** *This one literally makes no sense and it simply adds extra calories making it easier to gain weight and harder to lose it. Again, look at the reason behind the behavior. Are you bored? Are you eating just because it is there? Why? Fix the "why".*

___**"I have uncontrollable food cravings."** *Cravings are interesting because they can be composed of habit, addictive tendencies, food additives that trigger addiction, out of control thoughts, illness, sleep issues, and nutritional deficiencies. In other words, sometimes it's simply a bad habit, but it can also be a symptom of a bigger issue.*

___**"I crave sugar."** *Sometimes, it's just a bad habit. The subconscious part of your mind controls habits, so learning how to rewire your brain can be key here. Properly applied self-talk and hypnosis are excellent techniques for this issues.*

Sugar is addictive because it triggers the release of chemicals that set off the brain's pleasure center. Like drugs, people develop a tolerance and become sensitized to sugar, adding to its addictive nature. If this is the case, going "cold turkey" is likely the best way to go. However, as always, it's wise to look at why you might crave sugar, so that you may address the root cause.

How do you sleep? Often times fatigue can cause people to reach for a pick-me-up in the form of sugar. It can temporarily increase the illusion of having more energy, but ultimately fails and usually ends up making the person feel worse and more tired. Research has shown that poor sleep can impact your hormones. It can increase ghrelin (the hunger hormone) and reduces leptin (the hormone that allows you to feel satiated).

There can be physical reasons for your sugar cravings as well. Sometimes the root cause of sugar cravings is actually a nutritional deficiency, such as magnesium, iron, complex carbohydrates, and protein. You may want to have your vitamin levels checked, but meanwhile, take a close look at your dietary habits in general. Poor choices can easily lead to increased sugar cravings.

Another cause for sugar cravings can be the result of an imbalance in your gut health. Imbalances in the beneficial bacteria that inhabit the intestinal tract can lead to overgrowth of yeast and fungi. When you eat a lot of sweets, the bacteria in your digestive system end up feeding on the sugar in your diet, only making the problem worse with the more sugar you eat. These imbalances can create yeast and fungal overgrowth.

If you've had antibiotics or antacids, there's a good possibility that they've triggered an overgrowth of bad bacteria. Antibiotics kill off "good" bacteria and antacids neutralize the stomach acid that normally helps keep bad bacteria in place. Since the resulting yeast over-population feeds on sugar, it can cause cravings. Eating sugar makes the yeast multiply, thus intensifying cravings and creating a vicious circle.

To help restore your gut health, reduce or eliminate the amount of processed foods and sugar in your diet. In addition, add in probiotic-rich foods like sauerkraut, keifer, and yogurt, and supplement with a high-quality probiotic. Restoring the balance of bacteria can take up to five months, but with time sugar should become easier to resist.

Stress! Remember, sugar acts like a drug. It increases our levels of dopamine—the feel good hormone, so emotional eaters can be prone to reach for sweets. Additionally, stress can increase your body's secretion of the hormone cortisol, which can suppress your immune system, allowing yeast to run wild, causing almost constant sugar cravings.

We are all affected by stress in one way or another, which is why it's important to incorporate lifestyle strategies into your routine. Try yoga, meditation, exercise, or even just some deep breathing. The important thing is to recognize when you are feeling stress and separate feelings from food.

Hormones. Some women who experience sugar cravings associated to premenstrual syndrome are doing so because that is when endorphin levels are at their lowest. Again, we're back to the drug-like response. Menopause and perimenopause can also be the culprit as levels of the hormones estrogen and progesterone drop. As hormone levels change, the body tries to elevate levels of the hormone serotonin, and since sugar triggers a serotonin release, this can lead you to crave sweets.

Ironically, excess sugar can block your ability to turn GLA (gamma linoleic acid) into the DGLA (dihomo-gamma-linoleic acid) needed to produce prostaglandins that improve mood. If you cut out sugar, your body will make prostaglandin more effectively.

It's important to note there could also be underlying medical conditions that trigger the cravings. Thyroid problems, adrenaline overload, insulin issues, and diabetes can all be hiding in the background, and sometimes sugar cravings are your body's way of trying to alert you that there is an imbalance. If you have tried everything else, it may be time to get some lab work done to see if something is happening in the background.

___**"I crave salty foods."** *Like sugar cravings, sometimes it's just a bad habit, and retraining the subconscious mind can do wonders. However sometimes, strong salt cravings can be brought on by other things.*

Dehydration. Your body needs to maintain a certain level of fluids to function correctly. If those levels fall below what's needed, you might start craving salt as your body's way of prompting you to drink or eat more. Besides low fluid intake, **vomiting and diarrhea can** *lead to dehydration. When you're dehydrated, your body craves salt as a way to help you correct the imbalance.*

Electrolyte or mineral imbalance. Minerals help your body function properly. Sodium is a mineral. Sodium might not be the actual mineral your body needs, but the deficiency can manifest as a salt craving.

Lack of sleep. Again, lack of sleep can make cravings worse.

Excessive sweating. Sweat contains salt, so when a person sweats, their sodium levels naturally decrease. Excessive sweating is different than light sweating. Day to day or light sweating is nothing to worry about and fluids are easily replaced with water. Excessive exercisers or those who spend time in very hot environments may need to consume more salt to replace what is lost through excessive or prolonged sweating. Electrolyte-enhanced drinks may help restore balance to replace what is lost through sweat.

Addison's disease or adrenal insufficiency occurs when the adrenal glands do not make enough hormones that are vital for survival. People with this disease have salt cravings, in addition to other symptoms.

Stress. The adrenal glands are responsible for releasing cortisol. This hormone helps regulate blood pressure and your body's response to stress. Research suggests that people with elevated levels of sodium release lower levels of cortisol during stress. There is an association between levels of chronic stress, food cravings, and weight.

Again, ghrelin (which increases hunger) also plays a role here.

Bartter syndrome. Bartter syndrome is a genetic condition that is present at birth. People with Bartter syndrome cannot reabsorb sodium in their kidneys, which means that any sodium they eat is lost through urine, so they are chronically low on sodium, which leads to low levels of potassium and calcium as well. It can be managed with potassium, salt, and magnesium supplements.

Premenstrual Syndrome (PMS). For some women, food cravings for sweet or salty can be intense during this time. These cravings may be related to hormonal fluctuations. Not every woman experiences PMS symptoms. Women who experience PMS-related cravings may want to try taking calcium and vitamin B-6, chasteberry, or try acupuncture.

None of this is to suggest that you need to increase your sodium intake. In fact, some of you may benefit by reducing it. This information is to simply point out that sometimes the body sends us signals to alert us to other things.

___ **"I have fears about losing weight."** *Fears are typically revolved around past experiences or fear of the unknown. Sometimes people are worried they might be treated differently, or act differently themselves. This fear actually doesn't have anything to do with the weight, but is being generated for other reasons... reasons that are worthy of seeking out.*

Sometimes people fear losing the weight because they might gain it back. This fear is overcome by adopting a permanent lifestyle change, rather than temporary changes in food and exercise behaviors. If you have truly committed to losing weight correctly, then this fear becomes invalid. If you haven't truly committed to doing what it takes for a lifestyle change, then the concern is real.

___ **"I use weight as a form of protection."** *This is seen most often when there has been past abuse, typically in the form of sexual abuse. Somewhere in the mind of the victim, an idea of "I will be safe if I am less attractive so I will gain weight to be less desirable" begins to manifest. Years after the trauma, this belief system often remains in place, making it fearful to be thinner, in case it draws attention. When this is the case, the fear is a form of PTSD, and it usually involves acknowledgement and treatment to move beyond this barrier.*

___**"I do not exercise enough."** *Why? What is preventing you? You know the body requires activity. It's time to look deeper into what prevents enough exercise and start creating strategies as to how to overcome the barriers.*

___**"I am not sure what the right amount of exercise is."** *Is your body changing? Is it responding? If yes, then you are probably on the right track! If not, it's time to re-evaluate your approach. Re-read chapter 12.*

___**"I do not exercise consistently."** *Unfortunately, your body cannot store fitness. Some exercise is better than none, but without consistency you won't be able to properly interpret your own results and make adjustments to accommodate your body's needs. The best way to create consistency is to exercise daily, even if it's for a few minutes. The daily nature of it helps to establish it as a normal part of your day, thus developing consistency.*

___**"I do not exercise with the correct intensity for my goals."** *It can be tough to push yourself into exercise zones that feel uncomfortable with higher intensity than normal, but without the body being actually challenged, the body just maintains or degrades. Remember that the whole workout doesn't have to be intense, just interjected with enough intense parts to get your body to notice.*

___**"I am not sure what the right amount of exercise intensity is right for me."** *Is your body changing? Is your heart rate in the right zone? Re-read chapter 12.*

___**"I hate exercise."** *Then it's clearly time to re-think it. Exercise is needed. Your body was designed to move, so ignoring it's need for movement will lead to negative effects, rather than positive effects. But it's okay to be honest here. If you "hate" something, you won't commit to it as a lifestyle. So rather than forcing yourself to do an exercise routine you hate, start exploring different types of exercises and activities until you find what you love (or at least like). Would you rather work out at a gym or at home? Do you like exercise videos at home or would you like a group exercise class better? Would you rather exercise indoors or outdoors? Do you like simple or interesting approaches? Do you like to dance? Do you like to play pickleball? Hike? Bike? Martial arts? Be creative. It's about generating movement.*

___**"I won't make time to exercise."** *There' a saying that if you won't make time to exercise, you will have to make time to be sick. Proper exercise is the fountain of youth. If your health is a priority, exercise needs to be on the priority list of things to do. Find spare time by exercising while you watch TV or using part of your lunch break for a quick workout. The time exists. You just need to do some rearranging.*

___**"I am not motivated to exercise."** *Are you motivated to lose weight? The answer might be in finding exercise that appeals to you. Some people might find the treadmill horrific, but find great fun in playing racquetball. Other people enjoy getting sidetracked by the challenge of choreography in dance workouts while others enjoy the mindlessness of set routines. I used to love fitness classes, but now my favorite thing to do is ride my bike (well, it's a tadpole trike actually which is cooler and more fun, but that's just my opinion). Tastes change, so explore and adjust. When you find something you like and that works, it's far easier to be motivated. Forcing yourself to do workouts that you hate are not usually going to yield a long term commitment.*

___**"I do not drink enough water."** *Your body needs .5 ounces of water for every pound of body weight. Find creative ways to increase hydration. Any liquid that is alcohol free, sugar free, and caffeine free will count as water. Try herbal iced tea with stevia for variety. Try adding a water app to your phone or setting reminders to drink water. Buy a specific water bottle and try filling (and drinking) your particular water bottle up a certain amount of times each day to fill your goals. Your body will feel better, you will be less likely to overeat, you can curb cravings, and your body will be more efficient at fat burning.*

___**"I am not sure how many ounces of water my body needs to function well and lose weight."** *Your body needs .5 ounces of water for every pound of body weight, more if you heavily sweat.*

___**"I drink sugary drinks."** *Sugar is a troublemaker. Try going to diet drinks. Yes, they aren't the healthiest thing ever, but at least they don't add useless calories. No, diet drinks do not cause weight gain or sugar cravings and your body does not treat them the same as full sugar drinks. It's impossible. Still, water will always be a superior choice. Ideally, drink water or beverages sweetened with stevia or monk fruit.*

___**"I consume alcohol."** *Drinking calories is an easy way to gain weight. In fact, alcohol has more calories per gram (7) than carbohydrates (4).*

___**"I drink excessive amounts of caffeine."** *Less than the equivalent of 5 cups a coffee a day is manageable as long as you hydrate properly (no, the coffee doesn't fully add to the hydration number). Caffeine has dehydrating qualities (notice how you need to pee more when you drink it), so be mindful that you are not triggering dehydration which triggers cravings and overeating.*

___**"I do not appreciate and respect my body."** *Your body is amazing and it's constantly working hard to keep you moving and keep you alive. You are the partner of your body. In other words, your body is forced to deal with whatever you give it, good or bad. If you were to treat your body with appreciation and love, you would probably give it more of what it needs to perform well and look good. So ultimately, this is a cycle. Treat your body with respect and your body will reward you. Treat it poorly, it's harder for it to perform smoothly. Focus less on perfection, and more on appreciation.*

___**"I hate my body."** *It's okay to not be totally enamored by your current body. You probably have at least some discontent or you wouldn't want to change it via weight loss. Even when your body is in the* process *of losing weight, appreciation is needed here, even if your body is less than perfect. Once that healthy partnership grows, it's easier to tune into your body and work with it in a way that is perfect for you, and that appreciation and partnership may even grown into actual love for your body, which would be fantastic.*

___**"My relationship with my body is terrible."** *One step at a time. If your relationship with your body is terrible, then it's clearly time for a change, after all, this is the most intimate relationship you will ever experience. Like relationships can be, they can thrive or be terrible. Just like relationships, it takes two to work in harmony. Just like relationships, there's going to be good times and hard times.*

Have you ever been in a situation where you needed love, support, and understanding, but you didn't get it? Would it have felt better it you had? Think of your body in those terms. Your body needs love, support, and understanding. You are one with your body yet you are two different vessels, all at the same time. This relationship is unique and valuable. Once you start cherishing it, everything begins to change.

____ **"I don't understand my body."** *Study it. Learn it. Be your body's best friend and advocate. The more you pay attention to your body and its reactions (or lack of reactions), the more you will understand.*

____ **"I do not understand how to listen to my body."** *Your body is giving you feedback and information all of the time. Sometimes we get so used to outside information that we turn off the internal information. One way to re-train this, is to simply slow down and start paying attention. For example, the next time you drink a glass of water, notice how you feel before and after drinking it. Do the same thing with a meal. Do it again with a workout. Just start noticing. After a while, you will begin to notice the subtle and valuable information that your body will communicate to you.*

____ **"My "self-talk" is mostly critical."** *Learning how to become your own best friend and cheerleader can help you stay on track. Internal negativity can create defeat. Your words are powerful and create outcomes. Pick better words and create better outcomes. Re-read chapter 5 and start practicing positive self-talk, even if it seems a little awkward at first.*

____ **"I have issues with judgment and/or I think people judge me because of my weight."** or **"Other people can affect my weight or how I feel about my body."** *Once your relationship with your body strengthens and grows in love, you will discover that you no longer care about other people's thoughts or opinions on it because it's not their relationship! Your body is nobody else's business. They should mind their own. If someone is critical of your body, perhaps it's the relationship with that person that is the real issue.*

____ **"I sabotage my own efforts."** *Why? Seriously, ask yourself why. Is it fear? Is it lack of care? Why? Reflect. You know the answer.*

____ **"I have someone in my life that sabotages me or makes me feel unsupported."** *Sometimes this is intentional, but sometimes it's not. Either way, it should be addressed by having an open conversation about it and expressing what you need to feel supported. I have seen many cases where a spouse felt insecure when the other partner started to change their appearance. Re-assurance was what was needed here.*

When people team up to lose weight together, I have seen one weight loss "partner" sabotage the other based on their own frustration with their own progress.

I have seen partners and family members be outright insulting! I have seen people offer to celebrate a person's weight loss journey with pizza and cake. The list is too long for me to write out. The point is that sabotage or lack of support comes in many varieties. I would encourage you to talk to the person or people that aren't helping. Mind you, it's not actually their job to help (it's your body and your business, not theirs), however sabotage is not cool. Talk about it. If you are afraid to have a discussion with that person, perhaps there is something bigger going on. Ultimately though, it's your journey. Support is wonderful, but if you don't have it remind yourself that you don't need it! You don't need somebody else's support or approval to decide to change your life to be healthier. This gets to be about you.

___ **"I have weight-related parental issues."** *Many times people are still hurt by words that they heard or how they were treated in childhood. My own mom used to say I was fat compared to my sister. I wasn't actually fat, but I happened to have a very skinny half-sister. Regardless, it was an error on my mom's part, and she made a few errors, like we all do. I mentally resigned the insults to the "misguided quirks of my mom" file, and was able to love my mom dearly with no grudges or personal damage done to myself. But that was simply a technique I used. Basically, it was a form of forgiveness. Now I admit, had my mom continued that course into my adult life, she and I would have needed to have a conversation about what is in my "acceptable form of behavior / personal boundary" model. We didn't have that talk because it wasn't needed. In fact, the last time I was negatively compared to my sister, I laughed and told my mom that I didn't care if my sister was 30 lbs lighter than me because I was stronger and could probably bench press her! My mom just looked at me quizzically, and never said another word. Now I think that conversation was funny. Through forgiveness I was able to change the memory and feeling from one of potential hurt, to one that makes me laugh.*

People make mistakes. People can be rude or have weird quirks. People can say harmful things. Rather than internalizing the words and actions of others, let them own it themselves.

I'm not suggesting my method is the right one for you. But there is a way to heal from past or present comments. The point is to look for the healing and move on.

Nobody gets to decide what your relationship or goals with your body is... not even a parent.

___ **"My over-all confidence is generally low"** or **"I do not feel worthy. My self-worth is low"** or **"My self-esteem is low."** *These areas are important to consider and should be part of the weight loss process. While it's true that excess weight can affect confidence, it's also true that a sense of low confidence can affect weight loss results. A person with low self worth or self-esteem may internally feel as though they aren't worth the effort of weight loss and can be easier to discourage when they don't have a support system. In other words, they tend to give up easier. Mental well-being affects physical well-being. Work on the whole, not just the parts.*

___ **"I take care of others, but do not take care of myself"** or **"I am not a priority".** *Successful weight loss requires you to be on the priority list. Often times care givers or nurturers will devote all of their time taking care of other people or things and only give themselves the "leftover time" which rarely exists. Some people feel it's selfish to prioritize themselves. I think of it much like when you are on an airplane and you are advised to put on your own oxygen mask before helping others. Why? Because once you take care of yourself, you are in a better position to help others! Insisting on your own self care isn't selfish at all. It's loving. If you are healthy, you are in a position to help. If you are healthy, you are in a position to play more and do more things. If you are healthy, your quality of life can positively impact others.*

___ **"I am confused about which diet to follow."** *Re-read chapter 9. Stop dieting. Start eating logically.*

___ **"I can't get the diet mentality out of my head."** *Have you been on a diet before and lost weight? Did you gain that weight back? I am guessing yes and yes are the answers. In other words, you have already used your body like a science experiment and proven that diets fail. Plus, they make you half crazy!*

I recently worked with a man who "knew what to do" to lose weight because of his extensive dieting experience, so he told me flat-out he was not seeking nutritional advice and only wanted me to help with the psychological aspect. I gently cautioned him, but complied with the caveat that he let me know if he ever changed his mind and decided that he wanted nutritional help. For the first 2 months he was quite pleased with himself. He showed me his nutrition journal (which was all wrong) but he didn't want my advice so I didn't comment and would just ask him if he had any questions yet, to which he never did. Then one day he comes in for his appointment frustrated and discouraged because he had a "bad eating day" and gained some weight. He was also tired of feeling deprived. He was practically beside himself wanting me to 'fix' his subconscious brain to not make bad choices. I told him that I can't fix his subconscious brain if his conscious brain is confused about what good choices are. I explained that lifestyle choices are not the same as dieting and there was no such thing as "bad" foods as long as there was a strategy in place. He was finally willing to talk about foods from a logical perspective rather than a diet perspective. Ultimately, he found success once he let go of the old diet mentality.

____ **"Food feels like an addiction."** *It can be. Addictive behaviors usually have other components (like obsessive thoughts, bingeing, loss of control, etc.) and tends to be an issue of psychology. You might benefit from simultaneously working with a mental health care provider while undergoing your lifestyle transformation or using subconscious behavior change methods.*

____ **"I use food as a reward."** *Food is often used for social and celebratory events, but for some people the idea of "I deserve it" or "I'm going to reward myself" gets out of hand, and the next thing you know lots of little reasons become reasons to eat or drink extra food or reasons to choose foods and drinks that are more calorie dense. There are multiple ways of dealing with this issue. Some ideas might be to socialize or plan celebrations around activities, instead of eating or drinking. You could also find other ways to reward yourself... perhaps buy yourself something, take a bubble bath, get a massage, plan that something special you've wanted to do, or maybe even just take a few minutes to yourself to meditate or relax. There are plenty of non-food options. Write some down.*

____ **"I use food or weight as a punishment."** *I could write a lot about this one, but it can go off into countless directions, typically triggered by something that has happened in the past. This can be a symptom of a bigger, underlying issue that likely needs to be addressed with a mental health provider, or at minimum, some intense self-reflection and unraveling. You deserve to be healthy. Why would you think otherwise?*

____ **"I am not motivated to change how I eat."** *Keep a food journal for 3 days and then take an objective look at it. Do the choices you make support creating a healthy body? If yes, then what is it that you think has caused you to have a weight issue? If it's not food, it has to be something else. Sometimes it's beneficial to have a nutrition professional take a second look. If on the other* *hand, food choices are a factor and you still are unmotivated or unwilling to change what you eat, then you want your body to do what it cannot do, or you will have to be willing to potentially exercise for hours each day to counterbalance the food choices. Ask yourself if you are genuinely ready to lose the weight.*

____ **"I am not confident that I can lose weight or maintain weight loss."** *This is most commonly due to past dieting failures. Remember, this is not a diet. You might lose weight more slowly, as natural weight loss is slower than temporary weight loss. Therefore, you might need to be more patient and be willing to reanalyze how your body is responding to you and adjust when it hits plateaus (which are normal). Weight loss is possible though. You have to leave past dieting failure behind. This is not dieting. With a different approach, you should expect different results. Also, lifestyle changes are about longevity, thus creating positive results for long-term success.*

____ **"I think I am too old to lose weight."** *My oldest client is 88 and she has lost 112 lbs. so far, and is currently at the lightest weight that she has been in her entire adult life. She is just one example of many older clients that I have worked with. After a certain age, the approach has to be a bit different, but age is not the issue. Doing the right things (or not) is the issue.*

____ **"I want my body to change quickly, no matter the cost."** *The body can't healthily change quickly. Even weight loss surgery has a high cost, and I am not even talking about the dollar cost. "Quick" in the world of weight loss can mean damage to your metabolism, your liver, your kidneys, your brain, and your heart. Obviously, the healthiest way to lose weight is one in which your body can naturally process and respond to. I would deeply encourage you to look at the long-term picture. You will have fewer issues going forward, and find the journey to be much more peaceful.*

____ **"I am unsure what reasonable expectations and pace are for my body to lose weight in a healthy manner."** *The body can metabolize up to 2 pounds of fat per week if you are female and up to 3 pounds of fat per week if you are a man. If you have a large amount of weight to lose, these numbers may be higher. Remember, we are talking about losing fat… not muscle, not water… fat. Also, as a person who exercises, the scale can be misleading in terms of how much progress is being made. Measure your results through the number of bad habits that are being replaced with good habits. That's what allows you and your body to really change in more ways than just your weight.*

____ **"I have a health, hormonal, or medication issue that affects my weight."** *Nearly every health issue can be worked around. It's just that your approach may need to be customized for you. If medication is the culprit, talk to your doctor about other medication options or if there's a possibility of lowering your dose. Hormonal issues also present a change in strategy, but changing hormones do not doom a person to obesity. Bad habits do.*

____ **"I may possibly have a health, hormonal, or medication issue that affects my weight, but I am not sure."** *If you suspect this, write down any symptoms you may be having along with any questions and talk to your doctor. Maybe it's time for a physical, complete with lab work. It's a good idea to do this periodically anyway.*

Whew! That was a lot of stuff! But now that you know more about where you are, let's look at where you are going, and create a new checklist to track your progress.

READ THIS AGAIN

Food is necessary for survival, but food is not the intelligent being, you are.

Eat when you are hungry and stop when you are full.

The relationship you have with your body is between you and you.

Being <u>aware</u> is very different than obsessing.

It's much easier to control your fat intake and food quality when you prepare it yourself, not to mention much more cost effective.

Skipping meals can cause a downshift in metabolism.

Exercise is needed.

Your body needs .5 ounces of water for every pound of body weight. You are the partner of your body.

Be your body's best friend and advocate. The more you pay attention to your body and its reactions, the more you will understand. Your body is giving you feedback and information all of the time.

Your body is nobody else's business.

You don't need somebody else's support or approval to decide to change your life to be healthier. This gets to be about you.

There is a way to heal from past or present comments. Look for the healing and move on.

Mental well-being affects physical well-being. Work on the whole, not just the parts.

Successful weight loss requires you to be on the priority list.

CHAPTER 17

New You. New Goals. New Achievements.

Let's flip the old list into a list of goals and accomplishments. This list will also help you monitor your own progress and keep you aware of areas that still need attention.

This time, color in each box for each item. Once per month, re-check your list to watch your progress. Ideally, they will eventually be all colored in! Put an "I" to indicate areas that are improving, but aren't quite there yet. This list is a far better measure of lifestyle change than the scale will ever be.

Here's an example of what this looks like:

March 1	April 1	May 1					
				I am in control of food.			
	I			I can say "No" to food and mean it.			
				My portions are the right amount.			

Ready to start tracking your progress? Let's get going!

Date:

						I am in control of food.
						I can say "No" to food and mean it.
						I understand what correct portions are for me.
						My portions are correct.
						I do not binge eat.
						I do not binge drink.
						I eat in my own best interest and in the same manner, whether I am by myself or around others.
						I eat enough fruits and vegetables.
						I understand what the right amount of protein is for me.
						I eat the right amount of protein.
						I understand what the right amount of complex carbohydrates are for me.
						I eat the right amount of complex carbohydrates.
						I understand the difference between simple and complex carbohydrates.
						I generally avoid simple carbohydrates.
						I understand how much fat I should be eating.
						I generally avoid eating too much fat.
						I think about food only when necessary.
						My thoughts about my weight and body feel balanced and reasonable.
						Food is necessary, but I am not a food "addict".
						I only eat when I am actually hungry.
						My emotions have no association with food.
						Boredom has nothing to do with food.
						I avoid eating late in the evening or near bedtime.
						I eat out infrequently.
						When I am at a restaurant, I usually make healthy choices.
						I plan most of my meals in advance.
						I make sure that healthy foods are available to me.
						I can tell when I am full.

						I stop eating when I am full.
						I do not eat too fast.
						I can leave food on my plate.
						I avoid skipping meals.
						I usually get enough sleep.
						I avoid snacking between meals, unless I am actually hungry.
						I am free from uncontrollable food cravings.
						I am free from sugar cravings.
						I am free from salty food cravings.
						I am free from high fat and/or fried food cravings.
						I can lose weight without past fears.
						I understand what the right amount of exercise is for my body.
						I exercise enough for my body.
						I exercise consistently.
						I understand what the right amount of exercise intensity is for me.
						I exercise with the correct intensity for my goals.
						I have found exercises that I enjoy.
						I make time to exercise.
						I am motivated to exercise.
						I know how many ounces of water my body needs to lose weight.
						I drink enough water.
						I avoid sugary drinks.
						I consume very little or no alcohol.
						I avoid drinking excessive amounts of caffeine.
						I appreciate and respect my body.
						I am working with my body as a partnership.
						I am listening to my body.
						My "self-talk" is mostly supportive.
						I am unconcerned of what others think of my weight, because it's none of their business.
						Other people are unable to negatively influence my weight or how I feel about my body.
						I am free of self-sabotage.
						Nobody is able to sabotage my effort.

						Support from others is nice, but I understand that this is my own personal journey.
						I am free of being affected from weight-related parental issues.
						My over-all confidence is good.
						I am worthy.
						My self-esteem is healthy.
						I can take care of others if I choose, but I also take care of myself.
						I am a priority.
						I am not confused about which diet to follow, because I don't need to follow a "diet" to be healthy.
						I have let go of the "dieting" mentality. I am aware and logical with food choices.
						Food is not a drug.
						Food is not a reward.
						I do not use food or weight as a punishment.
						I am motivated to eat in a way that supports my goals.
						I am confident that I can lose and then maintain weight.
						I can lose weight at any age.
						I understand what reasonable expectations and pace are for my body to lose weight in a healthy manner.
						I accept and allow my body to change at its own pace. I have patience and understanding with myself and my body.
						I know whether or not I have a health, hormonal, or medication issue that affects my weight. If there is, I developed a strategy to work with it.
						Other: *(Fill in the box if needed)*
						Other: *(Fill in the box if needed)*
						Other: *(Fill in the box if needed)*

There is no doubt that my perceptions of weight loss are deeply embedded in a belief system of my own. Decades of experience in working in this area has given me very strong beliefs indeed. I have witnessed it in action and practical application over and over again. So it is not simply theory, whim, or the need to write this book that causes me to make this stand. I see it day after day, and it's a privilege and joy to witness the moments of realization when someone has a break-thru and success finally come to those who struggled so much before.

The keys to weight loss are how you eat, how you exercise, how you are, and how you think. When one of those keys is ineffective or missing, then all of the keys are ineffective for the long term. All of the keys need to be addressed in order to produce successful, significant, valid, and lasting change. The "keys" are the "whole" view of YOU and what you and your body need as a team to achieve the success you desire. When the keys are honestly and thoroughly addressed, then true weight loss success becomes the final outcome.

Obviously, this is not a diet; it's an approach. It's an approach which involves logic, patience, understanding, and love. When you apply those principles to your body, amazing things begin to happen for your body as well as your mind. This is about your whole self. It always was.

This is your personal journey. This is your opportunity to brave a new path with courage, knowledge, and appreciation for your own incredible body. Enjoy the process. Your body is a gift. All it needs is you.

Glossary

Aerobic – with the presence of oxygen.

Aerobic Exercise - exercise that increases the need for oxygen

BMR - Basal Metabolic Rate is the number of calories your body burns at rest to maintain normal body functions.

Calorie – A unit of energy.

Carbohydrates – an organic compound that occurs in food and that can be broken down into energy by people or animals.

Conscious Thinking – the component of waking awareness perceptible by a person at any given instant.

Diet - The kinds of food that a person habitually eats.

Hypnotherapy – a therapeutic tool for working with the subconscious.

Lactic Acid – A chemical produced in the muscles when glucose is broken down during strenuous muscular activity.

Law of Attraction - A metaphysical belief that "like attracts like", that positive and negative thinking bring about positive and negative physical results.

Macronutrient – A substance required for the normal growth and development of an organism. Macronutrients for humans include fat, carbohydrate, and protein.

Micronutrient – A substance, such as a vitamin or mineral, that is essential in small amounts for the proper growth and metabolism of a living organism.

Metabolism - The chemical processes that occur within a living organism in order to maintain life.

Neurobiology - The biology of the nervous system.

NLP - Neuro-Linguistic Programming is a controversial approach to psychotherapy and organizational change based on a model of interpersonal communication and the relationship between successful patterns of behavior and the subjective experiences.

Physiology - The branch of biology that deals with the normal functions of living organisms and their parts or how bodily parts function.

Positive Affirmations – Encouraging and supportive words directed towards oneself.

Protein – A key component of every cell in the body.

Reframing – Reframing is a language technique that causes a shift in attitude and responsibility.

Self-Talk – The words and thoughts running in your head.

Subconscious Thinking – The changeable, but automatic thinking patterns that controls most habits, beliefs, and perceptions.

Bibliography

Aerobics and Fitness Association of America. Reference Manual. Sherman Oaks: AFAA, 1994.

Alcamo, Edward. Barrons Anatomy and Physiology. New York, 1996.

American Council on Exercise. Aerobics Instructor Manual. Boston: Reebok University Press, 1993.

American Heart Association: Added Sugars. Retrieved March 18, 2019, from
https://www.heart.org/en/healthy-living/healthy-eating/eat-smart/sugar/added-sugars

Andersen, Charlotte Hilton. 11 Sneaky Things That Affect Your Weight That Aren't Food and
Exercise. Retrieved April 29, 2019, from https://www.rd.com/health/diet-weight-loss/factors-affect-
weight-gain/.

Atkinson, Lousie. Could Your Sweet Tooth be a Warning Sign That You're Ill? Retrieved July 5,
2019, from https://www.dailymail.co.uk/health/article-2042182/Could-sweet-tooth-warning-sign-
youre-ill.html

Bandler, R., Grinder, J. (1979). *Frogs into Princes: Neuro Linguistic Programming.* Moab, UT: Real
People Press

Berry, Jennifer. Reviewed by Elaine K. Luo, MD. What Causes Salt Cravings? Retrieved July 8, 2019
from https://www.medicalnewstoday.com/articles/319866.php

Branner, Toni. The Safe Exercise Handbook. Iowa: Kendall/Hunt, 1993.

CaffeineInformer. Top 25+Caffeine Health Benefits. Retrieved May 21, 2019, from
https://www.caffeineinformer.com/top-10-caffeine-health-benefits

DiSalvo, David. The Link Between Sugar And Depression: What You Should Know. Excess sugar is a
double whammy for your body and your mind Retrieved March 18, 2019, from
https://www.psychologytoday.com/us/blog/neuronarrative/201709/the-link-between-sugar-and-
depression-what-you-should-know

Donatelle, Snow, and Wilcox. Wellness: Choices for Health and Fitness. Wadsworth Publishing.
Oregon. 1999

Druckman, Daniel (2004) "Be All That You Can Be: Enhancing Human Performance" *Journal of
Applied Social Psychology*, Volume 34, Number 11, November 2004, pp. 2234–2260

Erin C. Hanlon, PhD Esra Tasali, MD Rachel Leproult, PhD Kara L. Stuhr, BSElizabeth Doncheck,
BS Harriet de Wit, PhD Cecilia J. Hillard, PhD Eve Van Cauter, PhD. Sleep Restriction Enhances
the Daily Rhythm of Circulating Levels of Endocannabinoid 2-Arachidonoylglycerol. July 8, 2019,
from https://academic.oup.com/sleep/article/39/3/653/2454026

Facty, Chris. Common Effects of Caffeine. Retrieved May 21, 2019, from
https://facty.com/lifestyle/wellness/common-effects-of-caffeine/

Gardner, Amanda. Soluble and Insoluble Fiber: What's the Difference? Retrieved March 1, 2019,
from https://www.webmd.com/diet/features/insoluble-soluble-fiber

Healthline. Why Am I Craving Salt? Retrieved July 8, 2019, from
https://www.healthline.com/health/craving-salt

Holland, Kimberly. Medically reviewed by Judith Marcin, MD on April 3, 2017. Everything You Need to Know About Hypothyroidism.
Retrieved April 20, 2019 , from https://www.healthline.com/health/hypothyroidism/symptoms-treatments-more#causes

How Much Body Fat Can You Really Lose in a Week? (July 18, 2007). Ehealth forum. Retrieved November 24, 2011, from http://kudosforlowcarb.blogspot.com/2007/07/how-much-body-fat-can-you-really-lose.html

Hyde, Cheryl. Fitness Instructor Training Guide. White Dolphin. Colorado. 1997

Hypnotherapy. University of Maryland Medical Center. Retrieved June 30, 2011, from http://www.umm.edu/altmed/articles/hypnotherapy-000353.htm

International Journal of Environmental Research and Public Health. Effect of Endrocrine Disruptor Pesticides: A Review.
Retrieved May 26, 2019 from https://www.ncbi.nlm.nih.gov/pmc/articles/PMC3138025/

Joseph, Micheal. Type 3 Diabetes: The Alarming Link Between Alzheimer's and Diet. Retrieved March 18, 2019, from https://www.nutritionadvance.com/type-3-diabetes-alzheimers-diet/

Knupple, Anika. Sugar intake from sweet food and beverages, common mental disorder and depression: prospective findings from the Whitehall II study. Retrieved March 18, 2019, from https://www.nature.com/articles/s41598-017-05649-7

Lopez-Garcia E, van Dam RM, Rajpathak S, Willett WC, Manson JE, Hu FB. Changes in caffeine intake and long-term weight change in men and women. *Am J Clin Nutr* 2006; 83: 674–680.

Lum, C. (2001). Scientific Thinking in Speech and Language Therapy. Lawrence Erlbaum Associates. Mahwah, New Jersey London

MacMillan, Amanda. 7 Dangers of Going Keto. Retrieved March 4, 2019, from https://www.health.com/weight-loss/keto-diet-side-effects

Mayo Clinic Staff. Dietary Fats: Know Which Types to Choose. Retrieved March 2, 2019, from https://www.mayoclinic.org/healthy-lifestyle/nutrition-and-healthy-eating/in-depth/fat/art-20045550

Mayo Clinic Staff. Dietary Fiber: Essential for a Healthy Diet. Retrieved March 12, 2019, from https://www.mayoclinic.org/healthy-lifestyle/nutrition-and-healthy-eating/in-depth/fiber/art-20043983

Mayo Clinic Staff. Metabolic Syndrome. Retrieved May 6, 2019 from https://www.mayoclinic.org/diseases-conditions/metabolic-syndrome/symptoms-causes/syc-20351916

O'Connor, Joseph and John Seymour (1993). Introducing Neuro-Linguistic Programming: Psychological Skills for Understanding and Influencing People. London, UK: Thorsons.

Osterweil, Neil. The Benefits of Protein. Retrieved March 4, 2019, from https://www.webmd.com/men/features/benefits-protein#2

Pace. G. (Host). (2009, January 5). Life After "Loser": Every Day is a Struggle. *Today*. Retrieved November 7, 2011, from http://today.msnbc.msn.com/id/28449267/ns/today-biggest_loser_on_today/t/life-after-loser-every-day-struggle/

Park, Madison. Twinkie diet helps nutrition professor lose 27 pounds. Retrieved February 19, 2019, from http://www.cnn.com/2010/HEALTH/11/08/twinkie.diet.professor/index.html

Piotrowski, Paul. Why Negativity Turns Your Subconcious Mind Against You. Retrieved July 22, 2011 from http://www.paulymath.com/2011/07/22/why-negativity-turns-your-subconscious-mind-against-you/

Roizman, Tracey. What Are the Causes of Sugar Cravings? Retrieved July 5, 2019, from https://www.livestrong.com/article/96983-causes-sugar-cravings/

Romanski, Beth. 7 Reasons You Crave Sugar And How To Stop According to a Health Coach. Retrieved July 5, 2019, from https://www.furtherfood.com/7-causes-for-sugar-cravings-and-how-to-stop-from-a-health-coach/

Scott, Jennifer. (2010, December 22) How to Calculate Your Caloric Needs and Lose Weight. Retrieved December 1, 2011, from http://weightloss.about.com/od/eatsmart/a/blcalintake.htm

Simpson, Terry. BMR Calculator. Retrieved December 3, 2011, from http://drsimpson.net/weight-loss/BMR-calculator.htm

Sorgan, Carol. Why Aren't You Losing Weight? Retrieved April 29, 2019 from https://www.webmd.com/diet/obesity/features/why-arent-you-losing-weight#1

Steinbach, AM., (1984) "Neurolinguistic Programming: A Systematic Approach to Change". *Canadian Family Physician*. 1984 January; 30: 147–150. PubMed What Percentage of the Mind is Conscious in Relation to Subconscious? Wikipedia. Retrieved August 2, 2011, from http://wiki.answers.com/Q/What_percentage_of_the_mind_is_conscious_in_relation_to_subconscious

WebMD Medical Reference Reviewed by Hansa D. Bhargava, MD on April 30, 2013. Is Lack of Sleep Causing You to Gain Weight? Retrieved July 5, 2019, from https://www.webmd.com/sleep-disorders/features/lack-of-sleep-weight-gain#2

WebMD Medical Reference Reviewed by Michael Dansinger, MD on November 14, 2018. Cushing's Syndrome. Retrieved May 1, 2019, from https://www.webmd.com/a-to-z-guides/cushing-syndrome#1

Westerterp-Plantenga MS, Lejeune MP, Kovacs EM. Body weight loss and weight maintenance in relation to habitual caffeine intake and green tea supplementation. *Obes Res* 2005; **13**: 1195–1204.

Winston, Courtney. What are Healthy Simple Carbohydrates? Retrieved March 5, 2019, from https://healthyeating.sfgate.com/healthy-simple-carbohydrates-6348.html

Youkin, Lainey. What is a Complex Carbohydrate? Retrieved March 11, 2019, from http://www.eatingwell.com/article/290631/what-is-a-complex-carbohydrate/

Index

Made in the USA
Las Vegas, NV
01 September 2022

54493832R00096